Dr. Albert Zehr's

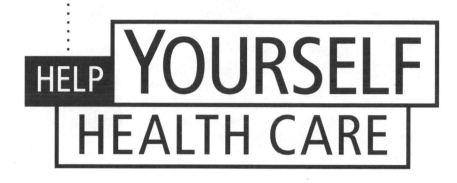

# HELP YOURSELF HEALTH CARE

Albert Zehr, Ph.D.

Abundant Health Publishers • Surrey, British Columbia

This book provides education and information which will assist the reader in taking positive action towardS better health. It is not intended to be used in the diagnosis or treatment of disease or to replace the services of qualified professionals. Any application of information in this book is at the reader's discretion and sole reponsibility.

*Help Yourself Health Care*

**Canadian Cataloguing in Publication Data**

Zehr, Albert.
  Dr. Albert Zehr's help yourself health care

  Includes bibliographical references and index.
  ISBN 0-9694418-2-7

  1. Diet therapy – Popular works. 2. Self-Care, Health. I. Title.
II. Title: Help yourself health care.
RM216.Z44 1997        615.8'54                    C97-910593-5



Published by:
  Abundant Health Publishers
  151-10090 152nd St., Ste. 531,
  Surrey, BC V3R 8X8

Cover Design by Caleb Chang

Printed in Canada

# *Dedication*

This book is dedicated to three wonderful men:

My father, **Ervin Zehr**, who became a "health nut" forty years ago. He walked the talk and lived almost ninety healthy years. His courage to be different and watching him dig his garden at eighty-eight inspires me to this day.

My son, **Ronald Zehr,** who not only walks the talk but also writes it. He is my editor, publisher, and friend. Without his tireless help this book would still be a stack of pages. I can't dream of a healthier relationship than ours. Ron, you're too great to be my son!

My grandson, **Anthony Zehr**, the healthiest, happiest, most beautiful product of *help yourself health care* and super loving parents. If other children could only be as blessed as you are. Thanks for letting your daddy help me.

# Content Summary

## Help Yourself Health Care

| | | |
|---|---|---|
| | Foreword | 11 |
| | Introduction | 13 |

**Part I  Understanding the Health Care Dilemma**

| | | |
|---|---|---|
| 1. | Health Care in Trouble | 17 |
| 2. | Changing our Perspective | 25 |
| 3. | The Devastation of Our Food Supply | 37 |
| 4. | A Paradigm Shift | 43 |
| 5. | Determining Your Life Potential | 61 |
| 6. | Determining Your Weight Potential | 83 |

**Part II  Good Health as a Daily Practice**

| | | |
|---|---|---|
| 7. | Getting Clear on the Basics | 89 |
| 8. | Nutrition – the Basis for Good Health | 93 |
| 9. | Food Specifics – What? Why? and How? | 103 |
| 10. | More Water Please | 119 |
| 11. | A Summary of Healthy Elements and a Place for Supplements | 125 |
| 12. | Elimination | 149 |
| 13. | The Immune System | 157 |
| 14. | Nutrition for Pregnancy and Pre-Conception | 163 |
| 15. | Special Concerns for Infants and Children | 169 |
| 16. | The Spiritual Dimension of Man | 185 |

**Part III  Health Problems and Natural Remedies**

| | | |
|---|---|---|
| 17. | Body Talk | 195 |
| 18. | Understanding Disease Categories | 201 |
| 19. | Diseases and Natural Therapies | 213 |

| | | |
|---|---|---|
| | Bibliography | 259 |
| | Index | 262 |

# Table of Contents

FOREWORD ............................................................................... 11

INTRODUCTION ...................................................................... 13

PART ONE: UNDERSTANDING THE HEALTH CARE DILEMMA. 15

1. Health Care in Trouble ......................................................... 17
   Early Warnings............................................................................. 17
   The Real Issues ............................................................................ 19
2. Changing Our Perspective ....................................................25
   Facing the Dilemma ..................................................................... 26
   Rising Above False Premises ......................................................... 27
3. The Devastation of Our Food Supply ....................................37
   Food Processing Disregards Nutrition .......................................... 38
   Setup for Malnutrition ................................................................ 39
   Animal Nutrition Superior to Human Nutrition............................ 40
4. A Paradigm Shift .................................................................43
   From Reactive to Proactive .......................................................... 44
   From Pain is Bad – Kill It To Pain is Instructive – Interpret It .............. 45
   From Symptomatic Relief To Symptom Interpretation ..................... 47
   From Drug Therapy To Herbal Medicine ...................................... 48
   From Compartmentalized To Holistic .......................................... 49
   From Immune Suppression To Immune Support ............................ 50
   From Chemicalization To Detoxification ...................................... 51
   From  Dependency To Enablement, Empowerment ...................... 52
   From Irresponsibility To Personal Responsibility .......................... 53
   From Passivity To Active Involvement .......................................... 53
   From Monologue To Dialogue ..................................................... 54
   From Suppressant To Facilitator .................................................. 54
   From Toxic Chemical To Phytochemical ...................................... 55
   From Antibiotic To Pro-biotic .................................................... 55

*From Synthetic To Organic* ..................................................... *56*
*From Monopoly/Exclusitivity To Cooperative/Alternatives* ...................... *57*
*From Taste Controlled To Body Response Directed* ............................ *58*
**5. Determining Your Life Potential** ........................................ **61**
*The Age Potential Profile – Instructions* ................................... *63*
*Concerning the Negative Factors* ............................................ *68*
*Concerning the Constitution Factor* ......................................... *79*
*Concerning the Positive Factors* ............................................ *80*
**6. Determining Your Weight Potential** ..................................... **83**

**PART TWO: GOOD HEALTH AS A DAILY PRACTICE** ................ **87**
**7. Getting Clear on the Basics** ........................................... **89**
*The A SED Theory* ........................................................... *90*
**8. Nutrition – the Basis for Good Health** ................................. **93**
*The Place of Nutrition in Human Health* ..................................... *93*
*So, What is a Healthy Diet?* ................................................ *95*
*Principles For Healthy Eating* .............................................. *97*
*Before We Eat – Time for a Healthy Pause* ................................... *99*
*Beginning With a Thankful Heart* ............................................ *100*
**9. Food Specifics – What? Why? and How?** .................................. **103**
*To Cook or Not to Cook* ..................................................... *104*
*What To Eat – Meat? Dairy? Eggs?* ........................................... *105*
*How Much? – Protein, Sugar, Fats* ........................................... *110*
*Food Combining* ............................................................. *115*
*The Body's Three Phases* .................................................... *117*
**10. More Water Please** .................................................... **119**
*Water as a Solvent* ......................................................... *119*
*Water May Be the Most Inexpensive Cure For Many Diseases!* .................. *120*
*Water Purification* ......................................................... *121*
*When To Drink Water* ........................................................ *122*
**11. A Summary of Healthy Elements and a Place for Supplementation** **125**
*Supplement Categories* ...................................................... *127*

Vitamins ............................................................. 127

Minerals ............................................................. 134

Fats .................................................................... 141

Carbohydrates ..................................................... 142

Protein ............................................................... 144

Enzymes ............................................................. 145

Phytonutrients ..................................................... 146

Herbs ................................................................. 147

**12. Elimination** ................................................... **149**

Two Aspects of Elimination ..................................... 150

Pollution is Everywhere .......................................... 151

Normal Detoxification ........................................... 151

Reduce Pollution Intake ......................................... 154

Practice Detoxification ........................................... 155

A Specific Cleansing Program .................................. 155

**13. The Immune System** ......................................... **157**

Numerous Lines of Defence ..................................... 157

The Workings of the Immune System .......................... 158

The Battle with Invaders ......................................... 158

Cancer and Autoimmune Disease .............................. 159

Care and Support for the Immune System ................... 161

**14. Nutrition for Pregnancy and Pre-Conception** ........ **163**

Preconception ...................................................... 164

Pregnancy ........................................................... 165

Smoother Labor and Delivery ................................... 168

**15. Special Concerns for Infants and Children** ........... **169**

The First Year ...................................................... 169

The Perfect Food ................................................... 170

A Nursing Mother's Diet ......................................... 170

(Almost) Every Woman Can Nurse ............................ 171

Dealing with Breast Infections .................................. 172

What if I Can't Breast Feed ...................................... 173

*Weaning* ........................................................................ *174*

*When to Stop Nursing* ..................................................... *176*

*Introducing Other Foods* ................................................. *177*

*How Often Do I Feed?* ..................................................... *177*

*Nutrition for Children* ..................................................... *178*

*Dealing with a Fussy Eater* .............................................. *180*

*Dealing with Sickness* ...................................................... *181*

*Vaccinations* .................................................................... *183*

*16. The Spiritual Dimension of Man* ............................... *185*

*Three Parts of Man* .......................................................... *186*

*The History of Man's Spirit* .............................................. *188*

*The Answer to the Dilemma* ............................................. *190*

*The Growth of this New Life* ............................................. *191*

*PART THREE: HEALTH PROBLEMS AND NATURAL REMEDIES* .. *193*

*17. Body Talk* .................................................................. *195*

*General Body Talk* ............................................................ *196*

*Deeper Observations* ......................................................... *198*

*Symptom Interpretation* .................................................... *199*

*A Further Step in Listening to Our Bodies* .......................... *199*

*18. Understanding Disease Categories* ............................... *201*

*Genetic – GN* .................................................................. *202*

*Allergy or Immune Related – AIR* ..................................... *203*

*Yeast or Infection Related – YIR* ....................................... *204*

*Thyroid and Metabolism Related – TMR* ........................... *205*

*Toxic and Environmental Illness – TEI* .............................. *206*

*Dietary Imbalance – DIM* ................................................ *207*

*19. Diseases and Natural Therapies* .................................. *213*

*BIBLIOGRAPHY* .......................................................... *259*

*INDEX* ........................................................................... *262*

# FOREWORD

*by Leonard Smith, M.D., P.A.*

As a physician and surgeon for over twenty years, I have seen firsthand the need to temper allopathic medicine with holistic practices. For the last 15 years, I have witnessed in my own private practice the dramatic progress made by hundreds of cancer and cardiovascular patients as they embrace natural therapies. I have come to recognize that without allopathy 20 percent of people would end up dead or maimed. However, it has also become more than clear to me that the remaining 80 percent of people can get far better help by learning and practicing the principles of natural holistic health.

Over the last several years, I have had opportunity to share the platform with Albert Zehr at a number of conferences. I have also had extensive discussions with him regarding natural health and have personally dialogued with numerous people who have received tremendous help from his lectures and writing.

In this new book, Dr. Zehr has created a wonderful balance. I was both inspired and educated while reading *Help Yourself Health Care*. In Part 1, Understanding the Health Care Dilemma, he clearly and poignantly describes the problems in our health care system and the shift that will be required and then ends with very practical tests for the reader to use to enhance their personal health.

Part 2 addresses what nutrition is, as well as the specific details with regard to food, water, elimination, immunity and supplementation. The third and final section of the book ties it all together with Learning to Listen to the Body and Diseases and Natural Therapies. It is appropriate that Diseases and Natural Therapies be at the end of the book. The message is clear: if one understands the first two sections and learns to listen to the body, the last part would never be necessary. But, for those in the modern world who refuse to slow down and listen, great benefit can be had from this last section.

In summary, I have great respect and admiration for what Dr. Zehr has created in this book. I feel all who choose to read it will be inspired, educated and benefited in their journey to optimum health.

# INTRODUCTION

Several years ago I met a wonderful couple in Pittsburgh. They were fatigued, overweight, discouraged and had nothing to look forward to but a retirement full of health frustration and endless medical expenses. A year later they declared, "Dr. Zehr you have totally changed our lives, health and future. You have given us back our life. We are now filled with energy, vitality, hope for many healthy years and a burning zeal to help others."

While I acknowledged their gratitude, I must honestly admit that they did for themselves what they attributed to me. I merely gave them the knowledge and the understanding to help themselves. That is what this book is all about. I have found that if people are sincerely willing to help themselves, they can "get their life back" and enjoy the healthy years that God intended. If you are willing to take some time and soberly and objectively apply the principles of *Help Yourself Health Care*, you can join the thousands who are in the process of keeping or regaining the good health which is available to all of us.

In recent years, I have lectured on the subject of health in over one hundred cities, in six provinces and twenty-four states. In all these places, I rarely find anyone who is assured that our present health care approach is on track and I have seen a dramatic rise in the interest in alternatives.

Year after year, audiences listen in rapt attention for hours, yet there is little evidence of behavioral change after the lectures. I have come to realize that we have all been deeply programed with a certain perspective. Until this perspective is changed, all that we hear is translated into the old and ineffective models. Everyone is really looking for a new "magic bullet" to replace the present unsuccessful ones. People expect new information to plug into the existing receptacles. We want better ways to force our bodies to remain functional and pain free, so that we can continue to ignore basic principles of good health.

Eventually, I have come to realize that unless we understand both our dilemma and how we got here, no fundamental change can take place. We do not need new ways which will merely propagate health failure. We need to see where and how we are on the wrong track. When we see the built-in failure mechanisms of the existing "health care" system, we will welcome change. From this new insight will come new understanding, which helps us to have both the will and the foundation for real change not only in perspective, but also in practice.

*Part One* of *Help Yourself Health Care* focuses on **understanding** how and why we are in a dilemma of misunderstanding which locks us into mediocre and poor health.

*Part Two* deals with the daily **practice** needed for maintaining excellent health.

*Part Three* puts forward natural **remedies** for numerous ailments.

If you are stuck with a definite illness, of course, you can go immediately to Part Three and see, "what to take for" your problem. If, however, you wish to regain and maintain daily good health, do take time to *understand* from Part One, and to *practice* from Part Two.

# PART ONE

# UNDERSTANDING THE HEALTH CARE DILEMMA

# Chapter 1

# Health Care in Trouble

## Early Warnings

Symptomatic expressions are the body's way of trying to get our attention. As the body becomes undernourished, toxic and exhausted, it begins to express its discomfort with symptoms such as aches, pains, swelling, rashes, or itching. If we don't make some adjustments, they will soon be followed by more serious problems. However, with no time to think and no knowledge to understand, we are programed to seek symptomatic relief as fast as possible.

The first question we are conditioned to ask is "What do I have?" It is amazing to what length sick people will go in order to find an answer to this question! From one specialist to another they travel, not resting until it is answered. What a relief when they are finally told, "You have 'something-itis.'" The assumption, of course, is that the answer to this question is necessary in order to find the answer to the next great question.

*... an increasing obsession with sickness rather than an appreciation for real health.*

*Part One*
*Understanding the Health Care Dilemma*

Now, the next great question becomes all important: "What do I take? Surely there must be a magic bullet that can relieve me of my disease. No doubt, the magic bullet will be specifically for the 'something-itis' that I have."

By seeking answers to these questions, we enter the system of what our western society calls "health care." Its real name, however, should be the "disease management" system.

Medicine has become obsessed with relieving symptoms. Success is heralded whenever a drug is found that can deaden pain, relieve an ache, or alleviate any form of discomfort.

*This assumes the body is comparable to an inanimate machine where parts can be separately adjusted or replaced.*

Eventually, simple medications no longer relieve symptoms, and more chronic symptoms are generated by the drugs already taken. Further discomfort and frustration now sets the stage for a quest to find answers to the resulting health breakdown.

The "what-do-I-have-and-what-do-I-take" approach assumes that diseases are lurking all around us and that for some unfortunate and unknown reason, some people catch them. When this happens, we must first identify the critter in order to know what bullet will be most effective to deal with it. Hopefully, if we

## The Drug Business – Dollars Without Sense

In the development of drugs, millions of dollars are spent in testing to determine what are the most effective dosages and the possible side effects. The drugs can then be patented so that the price charged will be sufficient to repay expenses and generate a handsome profit for the drug companies. This is why pills that may cost 10 cents to manufacture can be sold for two to five dollars each.

This is also the reason why vitamins and minerals or herbs can never get through this process. Since they cannot be patented, the cost of tests to satisfy the drug regulations can never be recovered. For this same reason inadequate funds are available to research and validate the efficacy of natural nutrients.

find the right bullet, we will have a cure or at least generate a temporary remission. Unfortunately, this approach rarely results in a cure. The assumption, then, is that there are no cures, and it thus becomes illegal to claim a cure for any major disease unless you are part of the disease management system.

Since there are no cures why not try to "deaden," "cut away," or maybe even replace the afflicted part – and so the disease management system grinds on.

## The Real Issues

Meanwhile, two crucial and far more significant questions remain obscured. Let's consider them:
- Why am I not well?
- How can I get healthy?

To find out the answer to "why am I not well?" we must investigate to see what is frustrating the body and why it cannot maintain its health.
- Why is my immune system unable to protect me?
- Am I toxic, depleted, overstressed, dehydrated, or exhausted?

The answers to these questions will then lead us to the second question, "how can I get healthy?"

This is what we will concentrate on in this book. The body already knows what the problem is even if we don't know its name. The body also knows what to do to overcome the problem. When we address the first question (why am I not well?) and respond with action to the second (how can I get healthy?), we are joining forces with our body. The body is then able to engage its self-healing capacities so that we can recover naturally. This is the way health was meant to be and this is the underlying philosophy of this entire book. This is the basic idea of *Help Yourself Health Care!*

*Unless we personally learn real self-help health care, our chances of reaching old age in good health are decreasing dramatically every year.*

### The Loss of Simple Health Care

Finding the best way out of a problem is often easier if we understand how we got into the problem in the first place. Let us consider the history of how our present approach to health care has emerged. Perhaps the following personal history will provide a number of crucial insights into how we arrived at our present situation of lost personal health care, and how we have come to be deadlocked into the disease management mode. These insights can be very instructive in helping us to understand the steps necessary to regain self health care.

*These insights can be very instructive in helping us to understand the steps necessary to regain self health care.*

When I was born in the late 1930s, my elderly Great-Aunt Barbara was midwife and care-giver. She had learned much from her great-uncle, Dr. Peter Zehr, who had moved to Canada from Europe, via Pennsylvania about 1825. While driving the horse and buggy as he made his rounds, she observed all his techniques. In addition, she learned through a lifetime of giving practical health care to many relatives and friends in the rural Southwestern Ontario community where we lived.

During my early years, Aunt Barbara's advice kept us healthy. If we did develop problems, there was the hot mustard plaster, hot goose grease, mashed onions, clay, or numerous herbal teas to facilitate our recovery. A fever was not something to be feared, but an integral factor in the healing process. Many times the advice was to just sweat and rest because a normal part of the body's healing was to "sweat it out." For a bee sting there was a cool mud-pack. An infected wound was soaked in hot milk. Mother knew the basics of keeping the family healthy.

The "real" doctor was available if the problem was very serious such as my older brother needing his half-torn-off ear sewn back on!

When I was nine years old, Aunt Barbara passed away, and it seemed like an era had ended. At the same time we moved to a new, more urban community. Almost immediately my mother was made to know that we had been living in the backwoods, even in the dark ages, as far as health care was concerned. Her new neighbors forcefully advised her that great progress in science and medicine had shown that those old remedies could not be scientifically proven, that much better health care was now available and that any responsible parent would be negligent not to consult the family doctor when any problem arose.

Mother struggled with feelings of guilt and promised herself that she would act more responsibly if any of her children got sick. She would not insist on sticking to her old ways but would be open to seek and take expert advice! She would never deprive her children of something better. Of course, she had never gone to college and didn't feel that she knew everything. So, why would she want to trust herself?

That same winter my younger sister and I both ended up with sore throats. Since this was a valid reason to miss school, we made the most of it with many moans and groans. This also afforded mother an opportunity to demonstrate her new determination to prove herself more responsible. So, off to the doctor we went.

After he looked at my swollen tonsils, the doctor mused that a tonsillectomy was in order. When mom asked what that meant, he realized that she was "medically illiterate." He simply assured her that if our tonsils were removed we would be less susceptible to swollen tonsils. When she asked why we had tonsils if we were better off without them, he simply advised her that since medicine has not been able to establish a purpose for them, they are best removed. He assured her that he knew what he was doing.

*Experience and tradition were not to be trusted.*

Medicine was now scientific and only what could be understood, or proven by double-blind study was acceptable. Experience and tradition could be trusted only if it was scientifically provable. Science had brought us far beyond those old ways. I'm not sure if he had double-blind studies to prove the value of tonsillectomies, but it was the "new modern way" and therefore acceptable.

My younger sister and I were ordered to appear at the hospital a week later and everything would be taken care of. We were assured that we would have less problem with sore throats if we had our tonsils removed.

After I awoke from the operation I told my mother, "I think this was a failure because I have the worst sore throat I've ever had." She assured me that the doctors knew what they were doing and this was best for us, even if we didn't understand.

My mother unconsciously was being conditioned to believe that health matters were too complex for her to understand. From then on, she became increasingly (and eventually totally) dependent on others concerning health care. Aunt Barbara's methods were somewhat apologetically used less and less while our self-confidence and intuitive wisdom gradually eroded. We eventually became another dependent entity in the "great wonderful developing" health care system which was based on science and in the hands of experts who were to be trusted, not questioned. Health care had arrived and there was no longer any need for us to worry, but simply to do "what the doctor says!"

*... unconsciously conditioned to believe that health matters were too complex for her.*

Twenty years later after being married and in the process of raising my own children, I awoke, as though from a stupor, and began to ask some questions.

- What was it that Aunt Barbara did?
- Are we really better off now?
- Why did we forget her methods so quickly?
- Were they just old fashioned superstition?

These questions and an irrepressible curiosity led me to careful evaluation and a return to natural health care. Eventually, I submitted a Ph.D. dissertation on "The Nutritional and Biochemical Dynamics of Numerous Folk and Home Remedies." In this research I did a careful in-depth analysis of many folk remedies (Native, Chinese, and Russian) to see if there was any scientifically provable basis to these practices.

I came to realize that these old remedies were very much in harmony with our body's innate, natural, self-healing dynamics. I also found that many of the remedies could actually be validated by science, but that there would be no significant economic profit potential in undertaking extensive research on them. I began to write and lecture on these matters and found that many people had experienced a somewhat similar history. In fact, I became convinced that my story encapsulates the health care history of North American.

From the story, we see how real health care was historically a matter of caring for and maintaining health by harmonizing with and enhancing the body's self-healing capacities. It was seen as a personal and home responsibility. In cases of injury, trauma or serious disease, the services of a doctor were used.

However, over the years, in a subtle, even unintended process, the entire care of our health became the exclusive territory of the trained doctor. Of all the professions, the medical doctor became the one who was not to be doubted or questioned, but rather trusted exclusively. Eventually, every sniffle, cough or especially every fever demanded a visit to the doctor. Results were demanded so the doctor had to do something. He had to give us something to take and thus, antibiotics and other medications came to be overused and abused.

Science was intended to seek and discover why and how things worked. In its zeal, it developed an aura of self-importance and gave itself ultimate priority. Eventually, no remedy was to be believed or practiced until science, according to its own standard of measure had determined its validity. If a remedy could not be scientifically proven, it had to be disregarded regardless how many centuries it had been used. If some "quack" insisted on promoting the remedy, it had to be declared illegal!

*Health care was historically a matter of caring for and maintaining health by harmonizing with and enhancing the body's self-healing capacities.*

Very often science has opposed reason and good sense merely because it could not yet prove or validate what was obvious to many. How many millions of people died of obvious smoking complications before smoking could "officially" be declared a health hazard.

The Shute brothers, medical doctors from London, Ontario helped thousands to overcome heart disease. But, since they used vitamin E, they were harassed and maligned and the use of vitamin E was mocked and withheld from millions whom we now know may have been helped by it. The same is true of Dr. Abram Hoffer and his use of niacin and other nutrients for treating schizophrenia. We could also cite the case of fiber for colon health and folic acid to avoid birth defects.

Recently, a new method of evaluation has been put forward. It is called "outcome based medicine!" The rationale is that since we can no longer afford to use the most expensive and most modern treatments, we should consider whatever gets the best results for the least money. Let a treatment be validated by the outcome of its use rather than whether or not it stands up to some legal scientific methodology. Wow! Isn't this how the rest of the world has had to function for years? Maybe there is hope.

*· knowledge*
*· practical guidance*
*· healthy choices*
*· natural proven*
*  ways*

The following pages will equip the reader with the knowledge for self-help health care. They provide you with practical guidance for daily healthy choices. For those with existing health breakdown, we will share the most successful natural proven ways to regain natural good health. While many will be primarily interested in Section Three, be aware that a lack of the knowledge of the material in Section One and Two is why the problems addressed in the third section developed in the first place.

I simply ask the reader to evaluate the theories and ideas of this book by the outcome of its application. If it works for you, as it has for thousands, then join in on the health care revolution!

*Part One*
*Understanding the Health Care Dilemma*

# Chapter 2

# *Changing Our Perspective*

*Note:* This chapter may be perceived to be negative and condemning of an honorable profession. It is not so intended. I have respected medical doctor friends who share many of the following views. Please consider the following as a sincere analysis of how we got into our present health care situation. In order to understand how to rise above a situation, a clear and objective analysis of how we got to where we are is really necessary. This can also motivate and inspire us to take action and help us determine what to do and how to overcome our dilemma. If this analysis offends you, skip it and move immediately to Chapter 3 which can stand on its own and still be very helpful without the following.

*Health and peace to you all.*

## Facing the Dilemma

*Health care in North America is in major trouble.*

Health care in North America is in major trouble and not just financially (although it will self-destruct in about ten years unless governments or someone find major finances really soon). An even greater concern is that it has strayed so far from its real purpose. It can hardly be called "health care" anymore. I call it "disease management" because all of its resources are being channeled into adjusting symptoms and helping people live with their sicknesses.

There certainly are many conscientious health care workers and many people do receive help. But, please allow us to take a sober look at the situation. I speak to hundreds, even thousands, of people who have been hurt, frustrated, confused and even kept in sickness by those who have been vested with the exclusive right to keep us well. In fact, current data indicates that one-third of the people in our hospitals are there and some will die as a result of medications and health care procedures.

*The time has come to face the present health care dilemma and to change our perspective.*

Those who perpetuate this system zealously guard their exclusive right to be the only ones with the authority to provide health care. As a result, others, including professionals from their own ranks, are prosecuted, de-licensed and labelled as quacks. These zealous efforts to maintain the monopoly of the medical establishment unfortunately also eliminates the need to become aware of effective options. Hopefully, the following points may shed some light to help find a way through the present impasse. One step in this process must be to expose and rise above the false premises which are a part of the platform of our present health care system.

## Rising Above False Premises

Consider with me how allowing the following premises to stand unchallenged may have contributed to a health care system that is often not free to put natural good health as its first priority.

### 1. Letting Science Control Rather than Serve

The twentieth century has opened its door wide to the world of science. What we saw through this door convinced us that science can give answers to every question and bring understanding to every aspect of life, especially concerning the human body and health. We not only assumed that science could understand everything, but also determined that it was the authoritative evaluator of all things pertaining to health.

This meant that any formerly accepted remedy or health procedure could only be regarded as valid or effective if it could be scientifically proven or validated. If science could not analyze it or understand and prove its efficacy by scientific methods such as double-blind studies, it could not be acceptable for an enlightened society. Furthermore, since science appointed itself as the guardian of truth, it saw fit not only to discredit what it could not understand, but eventually to disallow and forbid all health practices but what it credited as being "scientific."

Besides throwing overboard rich historical home remedies, medical science stifled innovation and greatly limited practical experimentation outside of its realm of control. No alternative health fields were given credibility and eventually all were made illegitimate.

All this set the stage to allow a monopoly the like of which has never been tolerated in a free society. Alternatives such as chiropractic had to undergo a mammoth struggle to gain access

*Besides throwing overboard rich historical home remedies, medical science has stifled innovation.*

to the public, and even to this day have never been given its due respect by medicine. An honest citizen who is able to help thousands to better health can still be arrested simply because he operates outside of the monopoly.

### 2. Health is Too Complex for Untrained Persons; They Must Depend on Professionals – Producing Total Dependency

*The consumer no longer takes an active role in determining the medical procedure.*

Certainly when critical matters of health such as acute disease, serious injury, surgical procedure and drug administration are necessary, they require highly trained professionals. The problem arises when the consumer is led, or perhaps even intimidated to believe that he or she cannot understand, let alone be capable of making, basic health decisions.

The consumer no longer takes an active role in determining the medical procedure. Rather then being given the alternatives and their various implications which allows active participation in reaching a decision, he is simply told what he must do. Sometimes it is even as preposterous as "You have X months to live if you don't take this treatment." While the gravity of a problem should be addressed, this approach disempowers the individual and destroys hope. It can be paramount to a death sentence. No one should presume to tell a fellow human being how long they might live.

A further tragedy arises in that the consumer, instead of becoming enabled and self-reliant, becomes increasingly dependent. Instead of learning how to regain and maintain health through nutrition and simple health methods (such as described in later chapters), the patient becomes totally reliant upon the doctor. Parents and individuals who should be trained to be largely self-sufficient are disempowered and become permanently dependent. For the sake of the health of our nations, surely, this matter should not be allowed to continue.

Parents in most other societies in the world know how to help their children through basic health problems such as flu, colds, earaches, fever, etc. But no longer so in America. Every sniffle or cough requires a doctor's attention, and, of course, the doctor must "do something." The doctor assumes that if the problem is bacterial, perhaps antibiotics will shorten the discomfort. If it is viral, antibiotics will have no effect. However, often, until recent public pressure forced a change in attitudes and practices, he would prescribe antibiotics anyway. At least he had "done something." These attitudes led to the colossal overuse of antibiotics and the devastating of the immune systems of a whole generation. They have set us up for a lifelong dependency on a self-serving health care system.

### 3. A System Where Profit Lies in Sickness Will Promote Health

In our society, money and profit play a central role in virtually all enterprise. It would be rare indeed for a profession to work against its own profit. Herein lies a major problem with the current medical setup. The money, the profit and the financial success are dependent on sickness not on health. When the surgeon decides whether an operation is needed, his income is directly and very significantly affected by his decision.

*Money, profit and financial success are dependent on sickness not on health.*

In every other area of society, we are very aware of and set up safeguards to avoid conflict of interest. How can a person whose income is very much affected by his decision remain fully objective! Perhaps the situation of firefighters might be consid-

---

### Heart Patients

In a study of 38,000 heart patients, those with health insurance (read that, the ability to pay) were 80% more likely to get diagnostic heart catheterization, 40% more likely to undergo bypass surgery and 28-48% more likely to receive balloon angioplasty.

---

ered a model. Their income is not increased by the number of fires they put out. Rather, a large part of their service is fire prevention.

According to our present model, the motivation to keep people healthy is certainly not inspired by financial consider-ations. Somewhat in jest I have suggested that a city council should directly hire doctors. They should assign them each a sizable annual salary to be paid in monthly installments. How-ever, each time someone in their jurisdiction gets sick, a certain amount should be deducted from their salary.

Almost immediately the doctors would be greatly motivated to research and study ways to keep people healthy and to keep them out of hospitals and free from drugs and medications. Nutrition and self care would become a central focus. Health care costs would probably fall and health status would, no doubt, rise dramatically.

### 4. Pain is Negative and Symptomatic Relief Equals Health Care

In normal situations, our body functions in a pleasant, pain-free manner. When it encounters problems, its immune forces immediately detect and analyze the problem and self-healing forces are engaged to enact recovery. In order to alert the host, the body engages a mechanism generally referred to as pain. Pain may express itself in various forms and discomforts, such as aches, rashes, swelling, eruptions, boils, nausea, etc. All of these are generally classified as symptoms, each indicating a deeper problem. However, instead of being trained and skilled in interpreting these symptoms, we have come to regard them as negative.

*Symptomatic relief has become the central and almost exclusive focus in health care.*

During the East-West Cold War, an early warning radar detection system was established all across the polar region of Canada and Alaska. This DEW (distant early warning) line was established in order to detect any threatening advances from the Soviet Bloc before they could inflict any harm to North America.

How foolish it would have been if America had focused on suppressing the DEW line, regarding its alarm as an undesirable factor in itself. Instead, even the slightest activity from the DEW line was seen as a possible indication of impending trouble and respected as a protective feature necessary for national security.

Again, consider pain or symptomatic expressions as comparable to the smoke or gas detection alarms installed to alert building occupants of impending danger. Now imagine a specialist trained in muffling or disengaging these warning devices for anyone who might be troubled by their annoying sounds. Eventually, such a specialist would try to convince consumers that alarms are primarily a frustrating annoyance and need not be taken seriously unless buildings are actually burning or people are already being overcome by smoke or gas. "…just come to us and we will give you a 'prescription' for shutting off alarms."

*See Chapter 4, page 45 for more on pain and symptoms.*

Hopefully these analogies show how our symptomatic relief focus is built on another false premise. In a further section we will cover the matter of interpreting pain and symptoms in order to avoid disease before it can make any advances.

## 5. A System Could Effectively Police Itself

Knowing the foibles and self-serving tendencies of human nature, democratic governments have always attempted to set up checks and balances to ensure accountability. Any organization should be able to be called into account by others who have no partisan interests at stake. This assures some degree of objectivity. It is particularly important for any organization which exists for the interest of the public so that it will not eventually use the public to serve its own interest.

*Any organization should be able to be called into account by others who have no partisan interests at stake.*

Most unfortunately this has not been the case in medicine. The rational seems to be that none but its own are competent to understand, let alone police, its activities. Consequently, medicine's own Medical Associations have total jurisdiction over the validity of its own precepts and the discipline of its own members. If members are accused of inappropriate conduct or improper procedure, the organization itself judges the matter.

The area in which this has been most detrimental is in the medical system's refusal to allow its members freedom for innovation. Certainly in such a serious science, there must be compliance to standards. However, through the years, numerous medical doctors who have conscientiously helped patients with unorthodox, unapproved measures have been seriously censured. I personally know competent doctors who have had their licenses to practice revoked simply because they honestly found that nutritional and natural methods served the needs of their patients best. Others have confided in me that they know that alternative methods would be more effective and less harmful, but are forced to compromise in order to keep their right to practice.

Only as the public becomes aware of the situation and demands that this system be governed by outside, objective interests and that access to all options be made available will this false premise be overcome.

### 6. Medicine Could Improve On or Bypass the Body's Self-Healing Capacities

*Whenever we think we can get ahead of or bypass the basic laws of nature, we begin to set ourselves up for trouble.*

This false premise is interrelated with the first false premise discussed above. Of course, science has learned much, but whenever we think we can get ahead of or bypass the basic laws of nature, we begin to set ourselves up for trouble. Sooner or later, we have to face consequences. Few would disagree that the body is self-healing and is designed to protect itself. But, then we try to take these principles and improve on them, speed them up or bypass them, because in our present society we have no time or patience to wait. We must have immediate results. Self-healing is really too slow.

To some degree we may be able to speed up or slow down the body's functions by introducing a foreign chemical, but we have not considered how this will affect the body's overall balance or future health. Countless people begin with a prescription to suppress a simple symptom. Eventually, the underlying problem and the drugs' side effects require more intense drug therapy and perhaps surgical intervention. The resulting drug dependency, debilitation and sometimes even early death may well have been avoided with a simple natural support for the body's self-healing capacity in earlier years.

No doubt, there are cases where direct intervention such as drugs and surgery may save or prolong a life. However, when this becomes the general rule rather than the exception, eventually the result is health chaos.

*We must consider – how will chemically altering body function affect our future health?*

### 7. The Human Body Can Be Compartmentalized

Realizing the complexity of the human body, it seems logical to compartmentalize it and study each part in greater depth. This allows specialists to focus on and to develop a much greater expertise in a given organ or area of the body. By now we have specialists for the eyes, ophthalmologists; for the heart, cardiologists; for the feet, podiatrists; for the brain, neurologists, etc. This specialization has its merits, but if the perspective of the whole is lost, problems will inevitably arise.

While the body is made up of numerous parts, systems and organs, they do not exist by themselves. The body is much more than a package containing all of these various parts. While each of the parts may be viewed separately, to deal with them in isolation can easily cause us to lose sight of the good of the whole. Eventually, each part is regarded as a part in a machine, to be adjusted or replaced at will. This can go to the extreme where the

*The body is much more than a package containing all of these various parts.*

operation is considered successful provided the immediate concern of the specialist was realized even if the patient dies.

Recently a certain cancer treatment was considered a success because it caused tumors to shrink even though the patients who received the treatment all died. The ultimate question which determines the success of any procedure must be the healthy survival of the patient, not simply whether or not the particular specialist realized his personal goal.

### 8. A Monopoly Works for the Public's Best Interests

This premise is probably just a further aspect of point number five above, but I believe it merits further consideration.

Since medicine is such a complex and highly technical science, it has been concluded that only those certified according to strictly defined criteria should have a right to practice it. It is further assumed that no one else should have any right to offer solutions or advice concerning matters of healing or even disease prevention for these are areas under the jurisdiction of the monopolistic establishment.

*Is it right that a certain group of people have an absolute monopoly over what is commonly referred to as health care?*

This arrangement has granted a certain group of people an absolute monopoly over what is commonly referred to as health care. Unfortunately, this has not only produced an inferior service, but also prevented anyone from offering a better option.

In all of this, the medical system has further been able to enlist the governments in promoting and enforcing this monopolistic stance. For instance, in Canada the federal Health Protection Act has what is referred to as "Schedule A."

Schedule A lists 49 common diseases and declares it a legal offence for anyone to claim a cure or a means of alleviation for any of these diseases. Medicine has declared them incurable and so they will remain until medicine in its own time and way determines otherwise. If anyone offers a remedy, even one that has a measure of success, for any of these diseases, he is immediately subject to prosecution. If any other industry was granted such power and absolute monopoly status, it would certainly become lax and inefficient in a short time. Why should we expect anything different from the medical system?

Of course, the rationale behind all of this protectionism is to save the public from false and harmful claims. But, the practical consequence of its enforcement has been that the best treatments for cancer and other serious diseases have been forced underground or to Mexico.

*The best treatments for cancer and other serious diseases have been forced underground or to Mexico.*

Meanwhile, in the United States, numerous medical doctors who have been successfully treating "incurable" diseases have been harassed, jailed, and driven into exile. Even in the 1990s clinics have been raided by gun-toting FBI agents and have had their records and property ruthlessly seized. The only crime committed was that they did not practice medicine according to the monopolistic rules. Hundreds of patients testified of remarkable recoveries. They were given no consideration, for how could the public know or understand what is best? Only those who hold the keys to the monopoly really know.

## 9. Nutrition as Found in Food is Incidental and Can be Taken for Granted and Supplements are Unnecessary

Diet and nutrition have been regarded as merely incidental rather than as an integral part of health care. Medical doctors trained in the 70s and 80s tell us that they studied very little nutrition, and assumed people were taught what was necessary in high school home economics class. Then of course, there were dietitians, those "experts" who planned the notoriously poor meals served at hospitals. Obviously these experts have been programed by those who have no awareness of nutritionally activated healing.

Many hospital patients tell me that one of their great

motivations to get out of the hospital is to avoid the lousy food. Several of our friends who have made extraordinary recoveries while at the hospital had supplements and nutritious foods smuggled in to them. According to *Nutrition, the International Journal of Applied and Basic Nutritional Sciences,* 43 percent of patients admitted to a hospital in Syracuse, New York were malnourished. At the same time patients in the hospital were receiving less than 60 percent of the nourishment they needed. Both of these factors were seen to delay recovery.

*With a little training and a little teaching, much sickness could be avoided and millions could enjoy a happier, healthier life.*

Without taking time to consider why this central pillar of good health has been so seriously neglected, we can only conclude that its neglect is costing millions of dollars worth of health loss. With a little training and a little teaching, much sickness could be avoided and millions could enjoy a happier, healthier life.

Since the above premises are fully ingrained in our present health care system, we can see that overcoming them is not a simple matter. It does, however, begin with awareness. Hopefully consideration and discussion of these matters will inspire many to work together toward real help yourself health care.

# Chapter 3

# The Devastation
# of Our Food Supply

At Expo 86 in Vancouver, British Columbia there was an Omnimax film on travel featuring everything from ancient travel modes to dog sleds to modern supersonic jets. At one point when a young boy was admiring the speed of a fast train, his grandfather remarked, "The faster man travels, the less time he will have." How true!

I remember as a boy on the farm in the 1940s when my father got a milking machine and my mother got a clothes washer. In each case, it was, of course, going to reduce the amount of time needed to perform those chores. Presumably, it was going to "make more time" available. Somehow, it didn't seem to have that effect in the long run. It certainly does seem that the faster we are able to do things, the less time we have! Not only do we have less time, but many of the important aspects of life are compromised, not the least of which is our health.

*In our hurry, many important aspects of life are compromised – even our health.*

## Food Processing Disregards Nutrition

One of the symptoms of this hurry-up, "no-time" mentality has been the fast food industry. This industry began even before the fast food restaurant craze. It began with the advent of food processing. In this era, convenience became king, while appearance and shelf appeal became queen. The former king "Fresh-from-the-field," and queen "Prepare-it-yourself" were dethroned, and King Convenience and Queen Appearance took over. Nutrition was largely disregarded.

*Prior to the advent of grain processing, colon dysfunction was almost nonexistent.*

Perhaps a classic case in point is the processing of wheat into refined white flour. Do you see how even the term "refined white flour" pays homage to the new king and queen? Before wheat is processed, it contains fiber to facilitate bowel regularity. In processing the fiber is entirely removed. Is it any wonder that prior to the advent of grain processing, colon dysfunction was almost nonexistent? The vitamin E necessary for a healthy heart and good circulation is 87 percent removed in refining while the remainder is destroyed in the bleaching process. Meanwhile, our medical scientists are desperately searching for a new wonder drug to cure the rampant heart disease and circulatory problems in our society! Many of these problems may be due to vitamin E deficiency.

*The vitamin E necessary for a healthy heart and good circulation is 87 percent removed in refining and the remainder is destroyed in the bleaching.*

Grains also contain protein, minerals, and other vitamins, all of which are necessary for good health. However, virtually all of these nutrients are stripped away in the refining process. So, for the sake of convenience and beauty, we end up with lifeless, bowel plugging, "dead bread" junk! This white flour is made into bread, cakes, cookies, and pastry – identical in nature and similar in function to the paste my mother used to make out of white flour. She used it for hanging wall paper. The innocent little children who are fed this junk, end up sitting on toilets straining to pass this stringy paste. When their eyes are dull and their faces pale from malnutrition, the parents may conclude that they need more antibiotics.

In an attempt to compensate for their wretched practices, food processors sprinkle an infinitesimal pinch of synthetic vitamins into the paste so that they can label it "enriched." Color it, give it fancy shapes and package it in beautiful boxes to be sold as nutritious cereal, which it certainly isn't! One would almost believe that the actual food value of the box itself is about equal to the contents of the box! And somehow we have been convinced that this is the best way to start our day.

## Setup for Malnutrition

Consider the following scenario. Children are awakened while they are still tired and exhausted and are herded to the breakfast table. In order to activate their appetites, they are given an attractive cereal – "dead" white flour, flavored, sugared and toasted then packaged in colorful boxes often with enticing trinkets. After dumping it into their bowls, the children pile on even more sugar and pour on highly processed, (homogenized, pasteurized) milk to which many of them are allergic.

*Many snacks leave children on a sugar high , but still devoid of nutrition.*

As they rush out the door for school, they are handed some "dead bread" sandwiches for lunch. When they return home after school, they are starving; so they eat twinkies, donuts, cookies or a chocolate bar, all of which leave them on a sugar high, but still devoid of nutrition.

By dinner time, their sugar-loaded bodies have no appetite, so they fiddle with their food. Dad gets upset and demands, "At least you are going to eat your roll before you can have any ice cream!" Eventually, nutritionally bankrupt, but filled with sugars and dead white flour, they go to bed, overfed but undernourished. The parents remind themselves to make another doctor's

*Parents remind themselves to make yet another doctor's appointment.*

appointment to see why their children have ADD (Attention Deficit Disorder) and earaches and are always catching colds.

Meanwhile, the barnyard pigs who are fed the nutrients which have been taken from the grains are much healthier than we are. Who said that pigs eat garbage? In America it's the people who eat the garbage; the animals eat the real food! Consequently, the animals in America are much healthier than our children.

*We have sacrificed nutrition and health on the alter of convenience.*

I have focused primarily on wheat. However, processing rice, sugar, and to a lesser degree, canned foods and prepackaged meals has the same devastating effect on nutrient content.

Some will no doubt reply, "We do not eat all that junk; we eat well. We eat vegetables, fruits and whole grains, so we are okay, right?"

While this is certainly much better, we must be aware that due to soil nutrient depletion and synthetic fertilization, even plants often contain far fewer nutrients than in the past. For example, you would need to eat more than a dozen bowls of spinach today to equal the nutrition contained in one bowl during the 1940s.

*One study found that lettuce grown in organic soil contained*
- *20 times the copper,*
- *90 times the iron,*
- *150 times the manga-nese,*
- *3.5 times the potas-sium,*
- *4.5 times as much calcium*

*as lettuce grown in depleted soil.*

Fertilizer used for crops essentially contains only three minerals: nitrogen, phosphorus and potassium. These three help the plants grow large with good color. However, the plants may still be severely lacking in the 10 major and over 60 trace minerals we humans need for good health. The fertilizer is applied for yield, appearance and profit, not for nutrition.

## Animal Nutrition Superior to Human Nutrition

A US Surgeon General's Report on Nutrition and Health states that diet-related diseases account for over two-thirds of all deaths in United States. Malnutrition is a real problem even in this land of plenty. Though we fill our bellies, our bodies go hungry. The processed foods and the crops grown in depleted soil cannot possibly meet our nutritional needs.

Upon visiting a sheep ranch in the prairies, I was informed that all the newborn lambs are immediately administered an injection of the mineral selenium. When I asked why, I was informed that this mineral prevents an otherwise common occurrence of white muscle disease, a form of paralysis. The farmers know that their soil is so deficient in selenium that the ewes do not get enough to protect their offspring. So, in the interest of better health (and in this case economics), the farmers give the lambs a supplement.

Meanwhile, we assume that the humans who eat plants from the same soil will receive adequate minerals. If our offspring have problems, we would never think to ask if there might be a mineral deficiency involved.

*Malnutrition is a real problem even in this land of plenty. Though we fill our bellies, our bodies go hungry.*

This could lead us into a lengthy discourse on how animal nutrition is far ahead of human nutrition. As a youngster on the farm in the early fifties, one of my jobs was to throw a small scoop of minerals on the cows' feed. Mineral supplementation has been used in animal food for decades, while human nutritionists are still arguing whether supplementation for humans is necessary.

Thirty years ago the preschool daughter of a friend of ours was having increasing pain and finding it difficult to walk. The medical diagnosis concluded that she was suffering from severe arthritis and that there was no way to help her. She was put in a wheelchair where she was to spend the rest of her life. She was told that her limbs would gradually seize up and lose their function.

*Mineral supplementation has been used in animal food for decades.*

One day when the veterinarian was attending to the needs of some of the farm animal, he commented on the child's condition. He had seen such conditions remedied in animals. Upon being questioned, he pled that it was illegal for him to treat humans, that he was trained for and restricted to animal practice. The mother insisted that he should at least tell her what he would do for an animal with such a condition. He said that he would assume a dietary deficiency, especially minerals, and would supplement the diet with minerals.

*Six year-old saved from lifetime in a wheelchair by nutritional supplements.*

The mother immediately began to administer this "animal" treatment to her daughter. Within weeks the child was on her feet, and in six months was running and playing as any healthy, normal girl would. Today, some thirty years later, she is an active career woman with high energy and good health.

Over time, her mother became a self-trained nutritionist who has helped thousands of people regain their health through nutrition. For years she was opposed and frustrated by "health care" professionals. Today, a number of medical doctors send their "incurable" patients to her.

The above story is a classic among many examples of help yourself health care which we have witnessed through the years.

Our modern society treasures convenience, appearance and instant gratification. When these values are placed on our food, however, the result is food that has been stripped of its nutrients. Even though we may eat abundantly, our bodies may still be crying for nourishment. Though our food may look lush and rich, on the inside it may be almost devoid of value.

While science and technology have done wonders with computers, electronics, cars and planes, our bodies are still made out of the same materials they were thousands of years ago. The more we treat them like our ancestors did theirs, the healthier we will be.

# Chapter 4

# A Paradigm Shift

Help yourself health care begins not simply with changing a few habits or activities. For many of us, it requires a significant shift in how we look both at health and at the so-called health care industry. We need a thorough change in perspective and a complete paradigm shift.

A paradigm shift involves looking at things from a different angle or from another perspective. Without a paradigm shift, things will always appear logical as they are and there will be no apparent need for a change.

The object of this chapter is to reinforce and elaborate on the concepts put forward up to this point. Until these principles are clearly understood, the probability of permanent behavior change is very limited.

First, study the list, then consider the explanations that follow. Try to comprehend their implications both for your life today and for your self health care in the future. Determine not only to learn or memorize each shift, but to fully understand and apply the required adjustments to your thinking.

To understand and implement self health care we need to make a shift in our thinking:

*From:* ■■■■■■■➡ *To:*

*To understand and implement self health care we need to make a shift in our thinking.*

| | |
|---|---|
| reactive | proactive |
| pain is bad – kill it | pain is instructive – interpret it |
| symptomatic relief | symptom interpretation |
| drug therapy | herbal medicine |
| compartmentalized | holistic |
| immune suppression | immune support |
| chemicalization | detoxification |
| dependency | enablement, empowerment |
| irresponsibility | personal responsibility |
| passivity | active involvement |
| monologue | dialogue |
| suppressant | facilitator |
| chemical | phytochemical |
| antibiotic | pro-biotic |
| synthetic | organic |
| monopolistic | cooperative |
| taste controlled | body response directed |

Now, let's look at each of these shifts individually. You may wish to explore and perhaps even develop these matters further. Here we will primarily elaborate on the existing model; the preferred models will be elaborated on in further chapters.

## *From Reactive* ■■■■■■➡ *to Proactive*

To be reactive implies a direct attempt to alter an already existing situation. In the case of a business, operating in reactive mode would mean that decisions are made and actions taken with little forethought about long-term consequences. The attitude is that we will proceed because it seems good for the moment, and if problems lie ahead we will deal with them when they arise. Any preliminary problems that show up will be suppressed or ignored until a serious problem threatens. At that time no efforts will be spared to directly attack and try to eliminate the problem. The problems that become crises may well have been avoided if a proactive or preventative mode had been employed.

*We proceed because it seems good for the moment.*

A proactive strategy would, on the contrary, evaluate all potential courses of action in view of their long-term consequences. Not only would the immediate situation be considered, but the long-term implications as well. During the course of progress, any minor irregularities, rather than being ignored, would be evaluated and addressed. In this way, serious problems would be prevented and reactive intervention would not be required later.

*... rather evaluate all potential actions in view of their long-term consequences.*

Surely, the application to health management is obvious. Yet, how seldom are the future implications of our daily diet and health style choices considered! Hopefully, the message of this book will help us to make a health care paradigm shift from reactive to proactive. The section on age potential should be of specific help in this matter.

*See Chapter 5.*

## From Pain is Bad – Kill It ⬛⬛⬛▪▪▬▬▬➡
### To Pain is Instructive – Interpret It

It seems that in health matters, we have declared pain to be the number one enemy. Having convinced ourselves that the essence of good health is to live a pain-free life, we have concluded that pain is bad, undesirable, and to be avoided at all costs. Since, pain is the enemy, we certainly should not tolerate it or dialogue

*We have made pain enemy number one.*

with it. If we cannot avoid it, we attack and kill it, or at least do whatever it takes to suppress it.

We must shift from such an attitude to the realization that pain is a messenger to protect and preserve us from damaging and destructive activity. Prior to any significant damage to our health, our body uses pain to attempt to alert us of impending problems. (This pain need not be acute or intolerable. It may be in the form of simple aches or discomfort.) Pain is a friend and a primary messenger. We must learn the language of this messenger, and respond to its message so we can save ourselves from more serious trouble.

*Pain is a messenger to protect and preserve us from damaging and destructive activity.*

It has been found that the destruction of the hands and feet of lepers is not the direct result of leprosy. Leprosy simply deadens the sensory nerves, so that the victim has absolutely no sensation of pain. A nail in the shoe, a stubbed toe, a blister, bruise or an infectious cut gives no pain and is not even noticed unless the hand or foot is carefully examined. The host, having no sensation of pain, has no awareness that he is abusing the weakened limb and deterioration takes place undetected. The messenger is no longer available and without its protective influence, self-destruction occurs.

*Learn the language of this messenger and respond to its message, so we can save ourselves from more serious trouble.*

None of us would choose to have leprosy. Yet, we aggressively pursue one of its symptoms. We determine to find ways to abolish the pain messengers, so that we can proceed unhindered with the destruction of our bodies.

For long-term natural good health, we must learn the language of pain and appreciate and cooperate with its protective friendship. If we interpret its message and respond with corrective measures, we can avoid future health breakdown.

## From Symptomatic Relief ➡️
### To Symptom Interpretation

Symptoms are the various ways that pain expresses itself. Itching, rash, swelling, aches, cramps, nausea, wheezing, coughing, boils, and blisters are just some of pain's symptomatic expressions. Having blindly concluded that pain is bad, symptoms have become unwelcome intrusions to be suppressed in any way possible.

Let's face it! When you have a headache, do you ask "<u>why</u> do I have this?" or do you ask "<u>what</u> can I take to get rid of it?" When you have a rash, do you ask "what is my body trying to tell me?" or do you persist in finding a cream or lotion to "get relief." Since relief is what we demand, the genius of science has been primarily directed to finding medications to be taken "for the symptomatic relief of . . ."

*We determine to find ways to abolish the pain messengers, so that we can proceed unhindered with the destruction of our bodies.*

How many of us have been taught to consider whether our rash might indicate a yeast overgrowth, an allergic reaction to a certain food or chemical, or simply a skin blemish that keeps popping up? Does the cramping in my legs indicate calcium deficiency, or do I simply need more aspirin? Is the heartburn I experience an indication of poor digestion resulting from bad food combining, or do I just need to take more antacids?

As symptoms are suppressed by drugs and medications, the underlying problems are not addressed. The symptoms become more severe, and stronger medications are required. In order for these medications to suppress the symptoms, they must in some way interfere with the body's normal processes. This interference often generates side effects, which also need to be addressed with yet more drugs.

*In order for these medications to suppress the symptoms, they must in some way interfere with the body's normal processes.*

Eventually, Mr. and Mrs. Senior end up in a nursing home taking a handful of drugs each day for a myriad of reasons.

Through the years, underlying health problems were allowed to fester. The drugs taken simply squelched the symptoms while the seeds of disease remained free to develop.

As health breakdown accelerates, an increasing number of their symptoms could no longer be suppressed. Many symptoms were deemed incurable and the victims were instructed to "just learn to live with them." Anyone who suggested there was a cure, or was so presumptuous as to offer an alternative, was written off as a "quack" and to be avoided. The professionals had decided that pain management was the best that could be hoped for.

Now in old age, Mr. and Mrs. Senior are reaping a harvest of disease and health breakdown. But, what if in their youth they had been taught to interpret pain, rather than merely seeking relief from it? What if they had had a paradigm shift?

### From Drug Therapy ▪▪▪▪ ▪ ▪ ▪ ▪ ➡
### To Herbal Medicine

*The consumers' desire for a quick and easy fix relegated herbalism to the fringes of public awareness.*

Since herbs have been used effectively since creation, scientists concluded that there must be some active elements in plants which affect the body's function. Through analysis and research, some of these active ingredients were identified and isolated. Entrepreneurs decided that if these elements could be isolated and chemical "copies" or synthetics made of them, these copies could be patented and sold as drug therapies. So began one of the most profitable and monopolistic industries in the world. Since this industry has been in total partnership with the medical profession, it has indoctrinated and totally controlled health care.

The aggressiveness of the drug and pharmaceutical industry, and its appeal to the consumers' desire for a quick and easy fix, relegated herbalism to the fringes of public awareness. After all, who had time to go out to the woods and collect herbs? And then, how were we to know which were safe and how to use them? Certainly no one should be permitted to bottle and sell them as effective remedies, even though they have been used for hundreds or even thousands of years.

*An interest in herbalism is spreading, bringing new hope to many.*

This "Drug monster" is developing a legacy of new diseases and drug dependency. At the same time, it is showing itself ineffective in dealing with cancer and numerous other diseases. While high finance and vested interests have blinded and held captive the health care system, some conscientious professionals and lay people have been awakening. An interest in herbalism is spreading, bringing new hope to many.

In my research on folk remedies, I found that herbs contain far more than a principal active ingredient. They contain numerous harmonizing and synergistic elements which cannot be duplicated synthetically. While drugs are invasive in that they invade and alter body function, herbs work in harmony with the body. Their primary effect is to undergird and enhance the body's innate healing and restorative functions. I have come to conclude that for every health need of man there is an answer in the plant world. Here again we need a drastic paradigm shift.

*Synergistic: the combined effect is greater than the effect of the individual parts.*

## From Compartmentalized 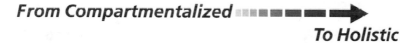 To Holistic

As knowledge increases, specialization becomes more necessary. This is inevitable because one person can no longer keep up with all the knowledge even within a particular field. So, today we have specialists for virtually every part of the human body – eyes, ears, nose, respiratory system, digestive system, blood, heart, etc. All the way from hair to feet – each part has become a field of study in itself.

*Each part is a field in itself. The holistic view has been lost.*

While this may be necessary, it has created a new problem which I refer to as compartmentalization. When any single part

*This holistic view further assumes that if the health of the whole is enhanced, then any one part will also be benefited.*

of the body becomes the of focus, it is easy to overlook the harmony of the whole.

The holistic view, on the other hand, insists that any one part must always be seen as merely a part of the whole. While in the broader sense holistic includes the spiritual and psychological as well as the physical, for our present purpose we are applying it merely to the physical. What we mean is that the physical body is one whole entity and a problem in any one part is a problem of the whole. This view further assumes that if the health of the whole is enhanced, then any one part will also be benefited. Conversely, if one part is not well, it suggests a deficiency of the whole.

In this regard, often when I am asked what to do about an ailing part or organ of the body, I respond, "How about we just get your whole body healthy, and then see if your specific problem remains? A healthy body is always willing and often able to restore its weaker members if it is given the overall assistance it needs. If your specific problem remains after your health is fine, then we will attack the specific problem." Eight times out of ten the specific problem will be overcome just by recovering good health in the ways we will describe in later chapters.

*Eight times out of ten the specific problem will be overcome just by recovering good health.*

## From Immune Suppression ▪▪▪▪▪▪▪➤
### To Immune Support

The body's immune system is an amazing defender and protector of our health. It is designed and programed to be precise in its detection of harmful invaders. Its destruction of damaging enemies in our body, and its ability to assess needs and prepare corrective elements for virtually every potential disorder are far beyond the understanding or capability of science.

When the immune system encounters an enemy, it develops specialized troops for specific antibodies to fight, overcome and rid the body of that enemy. After the battle, it will preserve the antibody "formula" for future use so that that particular enemy will have no opportunity to launch a significant attack in the future. At this point we say that the body has developed immunity to that enemy.

*The body's immune system is an amazing defender and protector of our health.*

As science has learned about the immune system, it has developed ways to activate it through the use of vaccinations. A vaccination introduces a small or weakened form of a particular disease. In response, the immune system develops resistant antibodies and easily defeats the weakened form of the disease. This immune formula is then permanently stored in memory, so that if the real disease attacks, the body can immediately resist. After a vaccination or inoculation, as it is sometimes referred to, we say that the person has been immunized.

*For more on immune system, see Chapter 13.*

While immunization has been unquestioningly hailed as a great breakthrough, it does have some inherent problems. To some degree, immunizations interfere with the immune systems intended work. This may frustrate and reduce the disease fighting ability of the body. (More on this in the section on children's health.)

*For more on vaccinations, see Chapter 15.*

My considered opinion is that most vaccinations, especially flu shots, are a waste of money and in many cases inflict far more misery than they prevent. In short, let the immune system do its own work in the way that it was designed.

## From Chemicalization ▪▪▪▪▪▪▪▪➡
### To Detoxification

Ever since it has been learned that chemical drugs have a significant effect on body function, the pharmaceutical industry has spent billions to develop drugs to alter body function. By now we have countless drugs to relieve pain, to reduce swelling and inflammation, to induce sleep or to activate or slow down heart

*The pharmaceutical industry has spent billions to develop drugs to alter body function.*

*Instead of introducing yet more chemicals, we would be much better off ridding ourselves of those already in our system.*

beat. All of this may sound exciting, yet it shows little respect for the body's own natural self-healing capacity. It also often shows a calloused disregard for the long-term dependency or damaging side effects that may well be worse than the initial problem.

At the same time that we are feeding ourselves with these foreign chemical substances, our bodies are being bombarded with more chemicals on the outside. Pollution and toxins are found in air, water, food, clothing, building materials, cleaning supplies, cosmetics, soaps – the list could go on and on.

The problems that supposedly make drugs necessary may well be the result of this myriad of chemicals and toxins in the body. Instead of introducing yet more chemicals, we would be much better served if we would rid ourselves of those already in our system. We should practice detoxification in order to relieve the body of frustration and allow it to perform its own self-healing function.

*For details on detoxification, see Chapter 12.*

Isn't it more logical to detoxify an overburdened toxic body then to add a further chemical load which can only exchange existing symptoms for new and more serious ones?

## From Dependency ▰▰▰▰ ▬ ▬ ▬ ➤
## To Enablement, Empowerment

If health care is to become the primary responsibility of each individual, we must break the circle of dependency. While the human body is complex and professional help is sometimes needed, the health consumer should become increasingly enabled and empowered rather than kept paralyzed in ignorance and dependency.

*Every time a person visits a doctor, he should learn something about his body and health.*

Every time a person visits a doctor, he should learn something about his body and health. He should be advised as to how to avoid future problems and what he could do to help himself. Instead, with each visit the consumer becomes more and more insecure and dependent, convinced that she can never help herself. Of course, part of this predicament comes from our society's acceptance of the medical profession as the ultimate authority in matters of health. If your child is to miss school, send a doctor's note. To validate your insurance claim, get a doctor's opinion. If a doctor says you need surgery, better have it done. If a health therapy is to be legal or not, ask a doctor. The doctor's word is sacred. Besides locking in dependency, this situation also sets the stage for the following points.

## From Irresponsibility ▬▬▬▬▬➤
### To Personal Responsibility

According to general thought, if a person gets sick it is nobody's fault, but if he doesn't get well it's the doctor's fault. If one doctor can't help me, I go to another who knows his business better.

*Take responsibility for daily life choices relative to diet and health habits.*

There certainly is a need to shift to an attitude of much greater personal responsibility. This involves taking responsibility for my daily life choices relative to diet and health habits. For this we need to become much more conscious of the health consequences of things around us and the things we take into us.

## From Passivity ▬▬▬▬▬➤
### To Active Involvement

"I went to the doctor, I did what he told me, and I took the prescription but it didn't work. If he doesn't know what I need, he should refer me to a specialist."

*This matter will be developed in depth in the following chapter on Life Potential.*

The above common attitude could be restated as follows: "I'm just a machine. The mechanic didn't fix me right. I will go back until he does. If he can't do it himself, he should refer me to someone who can, or maybe he'd best order a new part for me."

Our health is not something we passively hand over the keys to and pick up when it is fixed. True health requires that we ourselves are actively involved in its maintenance.

## From Monologue ▬▬▬▬➤ To Dialogue

One research study reported that the typical doctor interrupts the patient on average every 14 seconds. Obviously, the doctor is under time constraints since he works under a heavy schedule. Since the patient understands little about his own body and health in general, too much conversation or dialogue would be of little value. Time is better spent when the doctor does the talking. Hence, we have a monologue with no basis for active interchange.

Fortunately, more and more patients are beginning to take personal responsibility and rising up to take an aggressive interest in what concerns their bodies and their health. They expect to be informed and they intend to understand, give input and be involved in the decision making process since it concerns their health and their future.

## From Suppressant ▬▬▬▬➤ To Facilitator

*We must shift from looking for and employing suppressants to finding facilitators.*

The pain relief syndrome as described earlier focuses on interfering with and suppressing body functions. This overrides the body's natural protective and self-healing function. Over time, this kind of working at cross purposes with normal body function frustrates and greatly diminishes the body's own protective capacity.

We must shift from looking for and employing suppressants to finding facilitators. Keeping in mind that the body is always eagerly working to rectify disorders, we must find ways to help it. Detoxification can remove the frustration of internal pollution. Specific foods contain elements that facilitate the body's healing and recovery. Certain herbs stimulate and enhance the work of the immune system. To describe this, I wrote the following short poem.

"Can you heal yourself?" said the body to the injured thumb.
"Of course I can, I'm self-healing, I am not so dumb!
"Just clear away the garbage, cleanse the toxins and the dirt,
Supply nutritional power and I can deal with any hurt."

## From Toxic Chemical ➤
## To Phytochemical

A new word, phytochemicals, has come to the fore in nutritional concepts. It has been found that besides vitamins, minerals and enzymes, plants also contain very important plant chemicals. These elements, referred to as phytochemicals, are found in fresh ripened vegetables and fruits. One very important phytochemical called sulforaphane is found in kale, broccoli, cauliflower, brussels sprouts and turnips. It has been proven to be able to keep lab animals from getting breast cancer.

Tomatoes are a rich source of phytochemicals, including lycopene, and others which have been shown to destroy cancer causing substances called nitrosamines. A phytochemical called genistein, found in soybeans has prevented small prostate tumors from getting larger.

It becomes apparent that these amazing elements that protect our body and trigger and enhance body function are certainly worthy of much more attention.

*We must shift our concentration from chemicals which interfere with body chemistry to phytochemicals which work with the body.*

## From Antibiotic ➤ To Pro-biotic

The maxim "familiarity breeds contempt" is certainly true of antibiotics. By now, the overuse of antibiotics has led to the development of resistant strains of bacteria while at the same time compromised the immune function of countless millions. Since antibiotics are generally not very selective, they also kill billions of live and necessary bacteria in the intestinal tract. This allows fungus, like yeast, to run rampant. These yeast infections, such as Candida Albicans, greatly weaken the body's resistance to other diseases.

*Antibiotics kill billions of live and necessary bacteria in the intestinal tract.*

Antibiotics may also destroy vitamin K which is important for blood clotting and wound healing. When the viable or friendly bacteria in the digestive tract are destroyed, digestion suffers which in turn causes the immune system to be poorly supplied. The result is a weakened defence system which allows more infections which require more antibiotics – and the vicious cycle goes on. Friendly bacteria are also needed to manufacture the milk digesting enzyme lactose which helps to digest dairy products. The fact that these bacteria are frequently destroyed may be a significant clue as to why there is a dramatic rise in dairy allergies among children.

In contrast to antibiotics, there is an area in nutrition known as "pro-biotics" which deserves much greater attention. Pro-biotics such as lactobacillus acidophilus, lactobacillus bulgaricus, and bifidus are naturally found in the human body and necessary for proper digestive absorption but can be supplemented. When the intestinal tract has a proper balance of these friendly bacteria, digestion is effective, the immune system is keen and the body's disease resistance is strong. Supplementing pro-biotics should be considered as much more desirable than the use of antibiotics. For more on this see the section on the immune system.

*For more on the immune system, see Chapter 13.*

## From Synthetic ▬▬▬▬➡ To Organic

No doubt, one of the reasons why we are so often not inclined towards what is natural and organic is that life works relatively slowly and dictates its own conditions. So, we persist in finding ways to shortcut this tedious life process. Rather than going to the field to plant and harvest, we think to ourselves, "let's find a way to synthesize and mass produce a chemical copy of the real thing and perhaps we will get more immediate results. If the copy is identical in chemical structure, surely it will be effective. After all, the body will not know the difference, and look at the time we will save."

Sometimes I am asked: "Why is natural better for me? I have been told that scientists say both work equally well in the body."

My answer is simple. "If you were made in a test tube from synthetic materials then synthetic is probably great for you. If you were conceived by a natural biological activity and developed in a living organic parent then nothing can harmonize as well with your body as natural substances."

Scientists can develop "identical" sea water, yet fish cannot live in it. No creatures have ever been able to survive on synthetically produced food, and no life has been, nor ever will be, generated from a totally non-life source. No doubt, there actually is a Creator and his name is not science!

*If you were made in a test tube from synthetic materials, then synthetic is probably great for you.*

## From Monopoly/Exclusitivity ▬▬▬▬▬▬➡ To Cooperative/Alternatives

With all due respect to the medical profession's desire to protect the public from exploitation, the medical monopoly must be broken. Not everyone who offers alternative treatments is a quack or a charlatan. Not everyone who questions the present medical status quo is an ambitious, self-seeking rebel. Not everyone who is discouraged, depressed, unhealthy, and has been given up on by the system has an "it's-all-in-your-head" problem.

The betterment of the consumer, not the protection of an exclusive monopoly, must be the goal. To reach this goal requires cooperation, respectful dialogue and the consideration of all

*The betterment of the consumer, not the protection of an exclusive monopoly must be the goal.*

viable treatments. Discarding sincere questions with derogatory labels must stop, and a new era of cooperation must begin.

Fortunately, there are many medical professionals who are open to this dialogue. Some time ago I visited a doctor for a complete medical checkup. He went through all of the procedures as we engaged in active "healthy" dialogue. Rather than being threatened, he said, "What a relief to finally have a patient who does some of his own thinking."

Incidentally, he also said, "Although our visit has been inspiring, I must say that your test results are boringly normal, and with any luck I might see you again in a few years."

## From Taste Controlled ▪▪▪▪▪▬▬▬➡
### To Body Response Directed

*The question has nothing to do with the value of the food, but refers only to how it tastes.*

One of the first words we learned was probably "yummy." From then on our food experience primarily revolved around taste. The question we most often ask, "Is it good?" has nothing to do with the value of the food, but refers only to how it tastes.

Consider the statements we make relative to food: "Do you like it? That was delicious! I prefer it cooked. That's a good restaurant. What a feast! I could eat more of that." Are they not almost entirely relative to the taste?

Why does a person eat two large helpings of meat and gravy, then top it off with pie and ice cream? No doubt, they are controlled by their tastes and have no thought or awareness of their body's needs or requests.

*Our body wants to and can let us know what it needs and how much.*

It comes as a surprise to many to hear that our body wants to and can let us know what it needs and how much. In my lectures, when I tell my audience that our body wants to talk to us, I usually see some raised eyebrows. Finally, people admit that at least their bodies do tell them when they need to go to the bathroom. The sad fact is that we have never been taught to listen to our bodies. Except for the attention we give our taste buds, we are largely unaware and out of touch with our bodies relative to food.

If we would only develop a listening ear and a regular response, our bodies would gladly tell us what agrees with them and when we should quit eating. Have you never noticed how the relaxed contentment after a healthy, mid-sized meal turns into a feeling of bloating, indigestion and disgust toward food after you've eaten the dessert! Your body is trying to tell you something, but the taste buds are screaming so loudly and you are so used to hearing them that they usually drown out the "still small voice" of your body.

*For more on listening to your body, see Chapter 17.*

Having acquainted ourselves with the changes in perspective that are necessary for help yourself health care, we are ready to look at the effects that many of the things we do have on our health.

# Chapter 5

# *Determining Your Life Potential*

Scientists believe that the human body has a life potential of about 120 years. This has been confirmed in some areas of the world where people actually do live to such a ripe old age, many of them in a healthy state. This age potential is, of course, assuming ideal conditions, including proper food and a limited assault on the body's health. As we move closer to these conditions, we can expect an increase not only in life expectancy, but also in healthier old age.

People in our society generally have a much shorter life span by at least 30 to 40 years. The exercise in this chapter seeks to look at life potential in its relationship with many of the elements in our environment that may militate against maximum longevity. We must begin to see that day after day, everything we take into our body, or expose it to, very much determines our life potential. In other words, everything we do has a consequence. If only we could learn this while we are young!

*Everything we take into our body, or expose it to, very much determines our life potential.*

*Part One*
*Understanding the Health Care Dilemma*

*We all need a heightened awareness of the cumulative effects of what we eat.*

When I suggest that certain factors may be harmful, or frustrating to one's health, I am sometimes challenged, "Can you prove that such and such is harmful? Where is the scientific proof?" While the negative values assigned in the following list may be somewhat speculative, there is evidence for considering each of the corresponding items to be suspect. The overall value of the exercise should be a heightened awareness of cumulative effects. The greatest benefit should be in being inspired to reduce one's exposure to as many negative factors or stressors as possible.

The potential harm of chemicals is usually determined by testing them in isolation. We do not know what their effect may be if the body is exposed to them continuously or in conjunction with other elements. By the time we learn that long-term chemical exposure is harmful or that multiple combinations of chemicals are damaging, often the harm has already been done.

In a recent study of the effect of three different chemicals on mice, this problem was demonstrated. Individually, none of the three chemicals showed significant negative effects on the mice. But, when two of these chemicals were administered at the same time, the mice suffered some harm. When all three of the chemicals were introduced simultaneously to the mice, the results were fatal. This shows how, although the safety of a single item may be established, only time can prove what the effects will be in context with other elements. It is logical to assume that the elimination of any one of the following negative factors will decrease the overall stress on the body and thereby make it easier for the body to realize its highest life potential.

*Reducing the negative factors and increasing the positive factors will undoubtedly translate into a longer, healthier life.*

At the same time, we must become aware of and involve ourselves with health enhancing and life extending factors such as supplementation, detoxification, exercise, etc. Reducing the negative factors and increasing the positive factors will undoubtedly translate into a longer, healthier life.

The healthy life of my father generated in me the awareness

and the inspiration for this chapter. In his fifties, he became a "health nut," even before it was in fashion. He adjusted his diet and general health habits. Dad became the butt of jokes and was considered extreme by many of his peers and relatives. Yet, he outlived virtually all of them, not only in time but in quality of life. All through his eighties he hand tilled his large garden and provided vegetables for many others.

*My dad became a "health nut," even before it was in fashion.*

In his ninetieth year he finished his garden work and said he was more tired than usual and had lost his appetite. Two months later he spent his last three days in bed. On two of those days, he was still conversing with his family. He died peacefully in his sleep at home, as was his wish.

## The Age Potential Profile – Instructions

The goal of this exercise is to link activities with consequences and thereby inspire us to develop a sense of responsibility in our daily habit choices. Be honest when you calculate your scores. If you cheat you will be the only one who might lose something. If you take this seriously, we cannot guarantee that you will live a certain number of years, but we do guarantee a healthy learning experience.

*By making a few relatively easy changes, you might actually be able to increase your life potential.*

With a pencil fill in all applicable scores. Don't spend time to debate any point, just put down what is your first honest hunch. The scores are relative and are not meant to judge or convict, but simply to enlighten you on the possible implications of many things we take for granted. It may also increase awareness of the compounding effect of a number of minor "offences."

If you don't understand a point, refer to the descriptions and rationale beginning on page 68. If an area doesn't apply to you, leave it blank or put a zero on that line.

# The Age Potential Profile

**Name:**_____ **Date:**_____

| Item | Value | Explanation | Score |
|---|---|---|---|
| alcohol | -2 | 3 or more times per week | _____ |
| antibiotics | -1-2 | seldom to frequently | _____ |
| antiperspirant | -2 | containing aluminium | _____ |
| aluminum | -2 | cookware, foil, etc. | _____ |
| aspartame | -1 | regular use | _____ |
| candy/chocolate | -2 | once per day or more | _____ |
| chemicals at work | -4 | hair dresser, farmer, painter, etc. | _____ |
| cigarettes | -8 | any amount | _____ |
| clothes – synthetic | -2 | not wool, cotton or natural fabric | _____ |
| coffee, tea, colas | -2 | more than once per day | _____ |
| computer work | -2 | 3 plus hours per day | _____ |
| constipation | -2 | chronic | _____ |
| cell phone | -1 | 1 plus hours per day | _____ |
| dairy products | -1 | daily consumption | _____ |
| diarrhea | -2 | chronic | _____ |
| electric blanket | -2 | used while sleeping | _____ |
| fast food diet | -2 | more than 3 times per week | _____ |
| freeway traffic exhaust | -2 | more than 2 hours per week | _____ |
| fried foods | -3 | more than 3 times per week | _____ |
| fluorescent lights | -2 | work under | _____ |
| fluoride | -2 | added to water or toothpaste | _____ |
| garage adjacent to house | -3 | or under bedroom, etc. | _____ |
| gas furnace | -2 | hot air furnace | _____ |
| hair dyes | -1 | chemical base | _____ |
| high tension power lines | -3 | live closer than half block | _____ |
| high stress | -3 | routine lifestyle | _____ |
| | | *Subtotal* | _____ |

|                       |       | *Previous page total*            | _____ |
|-----------------------|-------|----------------------------------|-------|
| ice cream             | -2    | more than 2 times weekly         | _____ |
| margarine             | -2    | daily use                        | _____ |
| meat products         | -3    | 2 or more servings per day       | _____ |
| medications           | -2-6  | depending on potency/frequency   | _____ |
| mercury               | -2    | fillings in teeth                | _____ |
| microwave             | -2    | regular use                      | _____ |
| obesity               | -2-6  | 20 to 80 lbs overweight          | _____ |
| pill – birth control  | -1    | taking for more than 1 year      | _____ |
| processed meats       | -2    | containing nitrates, etc.        | _____ |
| root canals           | -1    | two or more                      | _____ |
| salt                  | -1    | added to meals                   | _____ |
| scanners              | -2    | work at checkout, etc.           | _____ |
| sexual promiscuity    | -4-8  | occasional to routine            | _____ |
| sleep deprivation     | -3    | chronic lack of sleep            | _____ |
| smoggy city           | -3    | poor air quality                 | _____ |
| soft drinks           | -2    | two or more daily                | _____ |
| water – inadequate    | -2    | less than 1 litre per day        | _____ |
| water – impure        | -2    | chlorine, fluoride, etc.         | _____ |
| work long hours       | -2    | average over 50 hours per week   | _____ |
| X-rays                | -2    | over once per year               | _____ |

If there is an inherent genetic weakness in your family history, such as diabetes, arthritis, heart disease, etc., are you taking conscious steps to protect yourself?  If not, count  -10                                 _____

*Negative Factor Total*                                                    _____

To determine **Negative Total**, take Negative Factor Total and if you have
a weak physical constitution multiply by 1.5                               _____
an average constitution multiply by  1                                     _____
a strong constitution multiply by  .8                                      _____

*Positive factors:*

| | | | |
|---|---|---|---|
| strong genes | +10 | parents both healthy | _____ |
| vitamin C daily | +3 | 1000 mg. or more daily | _____ |
| detoxification | +4 | fasting, or major detox biannually | _____ |
| fresh foods | +5 | 70% or more of diet | _____ |
| exercise – regularly | +5 | 3 plus times per week | _____ |
| supplements | +5 | multi-vitamin, minerals, enzyme daily | _____ |
| basic food combining | +5 | see chapter on food combining | _____ |

*Anti-aging researchers found the following factors to have a direct effect on the length of life of those who reached advanced years of life.*

For yes count +5, for somewhat count 0, for no count - 5

• Have you developed the capacity to accept, losses, tragedies, etc., and the ability to overcome and let go of fears, hurts, grudges and wrongs? _____

• Are you committed to and consistently involved in a long-term, positive cause, e.g. church, club, society? _____

• Are you active, mobile, on-the-go, walking, dancing, traveling, versus couch potato, TV, movies, reading? _____

• Do you have a positive attitude, seeing the bright side, full of hope and encouragement and optimism? _____

*Positive total* _____

Add: *Negative Total from page 65* _____

According to your present lifestyle, *your life potential score is* _____

## *Possible Score Values*

relative to age potential according to present life style:

| | |
|---|---|
| Above zero to -10 | 90+ years |
| -11 to -20 | 85+ years |
| -21 to -30 | 80+ years |
| -31 to -40 | 75+ years |
| -41 to -50 | 60+ years |
| -51 to -60 | 65+ years |
| -61 to -70 | 60+ years |

## *Explanatory notes:*

The object is to end up with the highest score possible and to see how specific changes could perhaps affect life potential.

Please remember the object of this exercise is not to debate the exact accuracy of the numbers or items listed. One could argue what is right or wrong or unreasonable about any item. Consider rather, according to your present lifestyle, what is your score? So, maybe you can't or won't change or give up certain practices. Probably, no big deal! But, it may be encouraging to see that just by making a few relatively easy changes, you can actually increase your life potential. What small or large changes could you make which could perhaps significantly affect your life potential? Those changes might just add ten healthy years or save you from five years of chronic misery, and that, eventually, could be a big deal!

After you have arrived at your score, look for ways and areas to improve by making lifestyle adjustments.

## Concerning the Negative Factors

### Alcohol – Three or more times per week                    -2

While there are some studies that indicate that moderate alcohol consumption may have some value, moderation is the key. Of course, there is also the ever present possibility of alcoholism. If alcoholism is a problem for you, better make your score a -5 to -10 depending on the severity of the problem. If you are not sure how severe your problem is, ask someone who can be objective and honest with you.

### Antibiotics seldom to frequently                          -1-2

*Until recent years, antibiotics were often prescribed even for viral infections for which they are totally ineffective.*

Besides killing harmful bacteria, antibiotics also kill friendly bacteria thereby setting the stage for yeast infections. They also compromise the immune system's ability to deal with bacteria and establish a natural immunity. Antibiotic use has become too routine. Until recent years, antibiotics were often prescribed even for viral infections for which they are totally ineffective. The overuse of antibiotics has resulted in the development of resistant strains of bacteria making the antibiotics increasingly ineffective.

### Antiperspirants containing aluminium                      -3

Any effective antiperspirant that keeps us dry requires aluminium as an active ingredient. Since it seals the pores of the sweat glands, the body is unable to release toxins in the way it was designed to. The toxins, then, must circulate in the blood or may even be held in nearby fatty tissue, such as the breast. This may perhaps be one factor contributing to the rise in the incidence of breast cancer. Furthermore, the aluminium content from the antiperspirant may be absorbed into the body and contribute to aluminium overload. A natural nontoxic deodorant is acceptable.

## Aluminium exposure from cookware, foil, etc.        -2

The aluminium overload connection with Alzheimer's and other forms of health breakdown is becoming increasingly evident. Any possible way to avoid it in food and water makes good health sense. Aluminium is found in antiperspirants, processed foods, white flour products, common table salt, antacids, and aluminium cookware.

## Aspartame – regular use                             -1

Time will tell for sure, but evidence is beginning to suggest that this artificial chemical sweetener may be a submerged time bomb. My hunch is that this is probably a -3, but I'll have to wait for more evidence. Frankly, I would personally use real sugar if I had to choose.

*This artificial chemical sweetener may be a submerged time bomb.*

## Candy/chocolate once per day or more               2

The dramatic rise in diabetes and hyperactivity parallels the rise in sugar intake. Refined sugar places a severe and unhealthy stress on the body's blood sugar control mechanism and adds stress to the immune system. Children who eat candy and drink pop have much greater incidence of hyperactivity, diabetes, colds and infections and require a much longer recovery time.

*The dramatic rise in diabetes and hyperactivity parallels the rise in sugar intake.*

## Chemicals at work (hair dresser, farmer, painter, etc.) -4

Some occupations inevitably involve the use of chemicals. If this is your case, there are some things you can do to diminish the potential harm. Detoxify your body regularly, as described in the elimination section of this book. Wear protective equipment, avoid direct contact and wash immediately upon exposure. Just

*There are natural alternatives such as vinegar and baking soda.*

because exposure doesn't hurt now does not mean that it will not harm your future. In the meantime, recognize the negative potential and compensate by a greater strictness in other areas.

The household chemicals used for cleaning and even deodorizing should also be a concern. There are natural alternatives such as vinegar and baking soda. Become familiar with them and do yourself and your family a favor by ridding your home of harsh chemicals.

### Cigarettes – any number                                    -8

By now millions of people have suffered great agony, remorse and premature death to prove what "health nuts" have been declaring for decades. As a child I heard a preacher define a cigarette as a deadly instrument with a fire at one end and a fool at the other. Before any teenager is allowed to smoke he should be required to spend several days in the lung cancer wards of a city hospital. Why would anyone want to gamble at a game where everyone loses?

*Before teenagers are allowed to smoke, they should be required to spend several days in the lung cancer wards of a city hospital.*

### Clothes – synthetic, i.e. not wool, cotton or natural fabric                                                             -2

While the evidence for this point may be inconclusive, allergic sensitivity to synthetic fabric is being seen with increasing frequency. This indicates that it does pose a frustration to the body's immune system. Natural fibers breathe and harmonize better with the body. Use them whenever possible, especially for undergarments and bed sheets.

### Coffee, tea, colas more than once per day              -2

The above contain caffeine which is an immune suppressor and if ingested on a regular basis frustrates healthy food digestion.

### Computer work 3 or more hours per day          -2

Computers, including the one I am working on this very minute, emit some level of electrical charges. Reduce exposure, by using shields, not sitting or having your face too close and taking occasional breaks.

### Constipation – chronic problem          -2

Regularity and a clean colon are necessary for good health. Be sure to get adequate fiber in your diet. If bowel movements are difficult or less than once daily, use prunes, bran, cascara sagrada, flax seed or some other natural aid.

*Avoid drugstore laxatives. Many of them contain sugar. Almost all of them stimulate the bowel by irritating it.*

### Cell phone– one or more hours per day          -1

If a cell phone has adequate energy to draw in radio waves, it can also affect the human body if held close to the brain for significant periods of time.

### Dairy products – daily consumption          -1

See pages 107-109 for negative aspects of dairy products.

### Diarrhea – chronic          -2

This can cause dehydration and inadequate absorption of nutrients besides indicating other problems which need to be addressed.

### Electric blanket used while sleeping          -2

Electromagnetic emissions so close and directly applied to the body have a negative effect on the body. If you must use one, use it to warm the bed before getting into it, but do not leave it on throughout the night.

### Fast food more than 3 times per week                    -2

Most fast food is
fried, high in fat
and sugar, and low
in general nutrition.

Most fast food is fried, high in fat and sugar, and low in general nutrition. This why it is generally referred to as "junk food." As an occasional stopgap measure it may have some merit, but as a general rule, it will develop a state of health frustration and malnutrition.

### Freeway traffic exhaust over 2 hours per week        -2

Sitting in traffic, breathing in the exhaust being spewed from the vehicles all around, literally makes us sitting ducks with increased susceptibility to a host of respiratory ailments.

### Fried foods more than 3 times per week                  -3

If you must fry, try a
quick stir-fry, but
better yet, go for
steamed or raw.

The high temperature required for frying destroys many nutrients and the fat used increases fat calorie intake. High consumption of fried foods often results in obesity and poor health.

### Fluorescent lights – working under                      -2

Fluorescent lights, except for the full spectrum variety, do not emit the complete spectrum of light rays needed by the human body. Also, all fluorescent lights release electric impulses. Be sure to work at least three feet from any fluorescent bulb during extended periods of time.

### Fluoride added to water or toothpaste                   -2

Fluoride, although not proven to be essential for humans, is found in plants, soil and animals. It is impossible not to get some in our diet. It has never been proven that adding fluoride to water protects against tooth decay. At the same time, it is known that excessive amounts are very toxic and dangerous to health. They have been linked to mongolism and Down's syndrome, as well as possible arthritic problems.

## Garage adjacent to house or under bedroom, etc.     -3

A garage is often filled with automobile fumes, including gas, oil and exhaust. Frequently, it contains leftover paints and solvents. If there is a door adjoining the garage and house or if the garage is under a room, it is inevitable that fumes will seep into the living quarters.

## Gas/oil hot air furnace     -2

A gas or oil furnace not only produces fumes from fuel combustion, but it may also recirculate toxic dust particles. Have combustion and ventilation checked and change filters frequently. A fireplace or poorly ventilated wood stove may present similar problems.

## Hair dyes (chemical base)     -1

Chemical based hair dyes applied to the hair are also easily absorbed through the scalp in very close proximity to the brain. Because hair does not have sensory nerves it is easily forgotten that it is a part of our body and should be treated as such.

*Chemical based hair dyes applied to the hair are also easily absorbed through the scalp.*

## High tension power lines – if live closer than half block     -3

High tension power lines are the ultimate in electromagnetic pollution. Just drive under them with your radio on and you will know that some powerful influence is at work. Persons with weakened immune systems should definitely not live closer than a block away from them.

## High stress routine lifestyle     -3

It has been proven that stress overworks the adrenal glands and decreases the effectiveness of the immune system so that the

*To reduce the detrimental effects of stress, be sure to take additional Vitamin C, at least 2000 mg. daily.*

body cannot protect itself adequately. Linus Pauling's research showed that if a goat is under stress, it greatly increases its vitamin C (ascorbic acid) production. Since we do not make our own, we should be sure to take additional vitamin C (at least 2000 mg. daily) to reduce the detrimental effects of stress.

### Ice cream more than 2 times weekly                    -2

Here is the classic case of a dietary no-no in the most tasty appetizing form – high fat with loads of sugar and protein. What a taste delight and what a digestive nightmare! And to think that we often throw it on top of a reasonably good meal. One lady we know insists that it helps her regularity. No wonder, her body wants to get rid of this garbage as soon as possible! If you must indulge, take it by itself in moderate amounts and no more than twice a week as a special treat.

*Make your own frozen treat with a blender.*

Try frozen yogurt or, better yet, make your own frozen treat with a blender. Try frozen fruit, with fruit juice or milk, frozen ripe bananas, maple syrup or honey as a sweetener, with ice cubes and blend to taste.

### Margarine used daily                    -2

Forget the margarine versus butter arguments. Neither are good for you, although butter is better. Don't touch fake fat or margarine, and use butter sparingly.

### Meat products – 2 or more servings per day                    -3

*Eat meat not more than once a day.*

My research, observations, and personal experience convince me that meat products are not necessary for good health and anything beyond a moderate amount has a negative impact on good health. If you choose to eat meat, take a small portion, about a third to half of the usual portion. Eat it not more than once a day. Taste it. Savor it. Chew and enjoy it, but don't indulge in it. You will be healthier without it.

## Medications depends on potency/time                    -2-6

Medications are a double-edged sword to say the least. While in extreme conditions they may extend life, their propensity to reduce life span is far greater. They should be used only as a last resort. Medications always have some detrimental effect and, if taken continuously, inevitably lead to a need for more medications as well as potential addictions. If you are taking medications, determine to find natural ways to generate natural healing. Countless people have gotten off medications by following the principles outlined in this book.

*Medications are a double-edged sword.*

## Mercury "silver" fillings in teeth                    -2

The silver fillings in teeth actually contain little silver. Their main ingredient is mercury. When they were first proposed, dentists were outraged. Who would think of putting a highly toxic heavy metal in a person's mouth as a permanent fixture? After it was shown that it was reasonably stable if mixed with other alloys and that it was the most economical and easiest to apply, mercury or amalgam fillings soon became standard procedure.

The dental association, against mounting evidence to the contrary, still insists that mercury fillings are harmless. They have finally acknowledged that some highly mercury-sensitive persons might be allergic to mercury and should consider alternative fillings.

Today, there is a large amount of evidence that the mercury may leech out of the filling, and an increasing number of immune breakdown cases are being traced to mercury toxicity. I know an increasing number of persons whose health frustrations were

*The dental association, against mounting evidence to the contrary, still insists that mercury fillings are harmless.*

relieved when they had the mercury removed from their teeth. This must be done with great care and by a specially trained dentist. I strongly urge all adults and especially children to choose alternatives if fillings are required. In some countries mercury fillings are already being banned.

### Microwave regular use                                    -2

*Microwaves change the structure of food.*

I am not really sure about this one, but this method of heating food is certainly not a natural process. Although few studies have been done, there is some undeniable evidence that strongly suggests that microwaves negatively change the molecular structure of food. These changes can encourage precancerous growths or disrupt the normal operation of various body systems and processes.

### Obesity – 20 to 80 pounds overweight            -2-8

There is certainly no doubt that excess weight reduces life expectancy. For more on ways to overcome this problem see Chapters 6 and 19.

### Pill – birth control if taken for more than 1 year       -1

The "pill" does have some negative effects on the body. If there is a long-term need for birth control, consider natural methods. Some of these have a proven track record.

### Processed meats containing nitrates, etc.              -2

When it comes to hideouts for preservatives, nitrates, nitrites and other suspicious additives – processed meats are the winners. If a mother would see the grey meatless waste which is turned into baloney and weiners simply by adding color, preservatives and flavoring she would never feed it to her cat, let alone her child.

Dog food is far more nutritious and safer than virtually any processed meat! Feed your dog or cat processed meat approved for human consumption instead of pet food, and they will live only half as long.

### Root canals, two or more                                    -1

Recent evidence points to root canals having some negative effect on the health of sensitive people.

### Salt added to meals                                         -1

While the body requires sodium, any excess amount can compete with potassium absorption and cause a potassium deficiency. Potassium deficiency is implicated in heart disease. There is adequate salt found naturally in foods. Adding more is unnecessary and may be dangerous. If you think foods taste bland without salt, go without it for two months. By then food will taste better without it.

*There is adequate salt found naturally in foods.*

### Scanners at checkout cash register, etc.                    -2

Similar to computer emissions. See section above on computer work.

### Sexual promiscuity – occasional to routine            -4-8

Since we are here considering age potential, we will not address moral aspects. From strictly an objective stance, there is no doubt that any form of sexual activity beyond marital monogamy poses an added degree of risk. The risk to health increases with the level and range of both sexual activity and sexual orientation and has been proven to have a very significant effect on life potential.

### Sleep depravation – chronic lack of sleep                    -3

While the amount of sleep needed does vary, any consistent lack of adequate sleep takes a toll on health. It has been shown that immune function and the body's ability to rebuild itself are decreased when inadequate rest is realized. For some the deterioration is gradual, for others the result may come suddenly with a physical breakdown.

*Sleep is the time when the body rebuilds, rejuvenates and heals damaged tissue.*

A recent increase in chronic fatigue syndrome and in fibromyalgia is being linked to chronic lack of adequate rest. Sleep is the time when the body rebuilds, rejuvenates and heals damaged tissue. If adequate time is not allowed consistently, deterioration and aging will accelerate.

### Smoggy city with poor air quality                    -3

The consistent breathing of polluted air is definitely related to a rise in respiratory problems. If you can't escape, take additional precautions in other areas. Also, consider extra air filtration such as an ion generator in your home.

### Soft drinks – two or more daily                    -2

Soft drinks are not an adequate replacement for water although many people drink far more pop than water. Soft drinks are laced with potentially toxic chemicals. They result in a net loss in fluid, not a gain, as the body tries to flush them out. Isn't it strange how we are concerned about pure water while at the same time we pay others to pollute our water for us!

### Water – inadequate drinking – less than 1 litre per day                    -2

Water is not only the body's cooling fluid, it is also the internal cleansing agent, as well as the vehicle which conveys all nutrients into the body. Most persons could improve their health significantly simply by drinking at least two liters of water per day.

### Water – impure – containing chlorine, fluoride, etc.  -2

Fluoride, a deadly poison added to water presumably to reduce tooth decay, will eventually be seen as a senseless health destroyer. Chlorine, while perhaps valuable for killing bacteria, also has been proven to be destructive. Chlorine can destroy polyunsaturated fatty acids and vitamin E and generates toxins which are capable of free radical damage. It also destroys intestinal flora.

### Work long hours – average over 50 hours          -2

The body has an amazing capacity for output, but it also requires time for input, restoration, rebuilding and recreation.

*The body requires time for input, restoration, re building and recreation.*

### X-rays more than once per year                    -2

As in so many other areas, experts have determined a safe level of exposure to x-rays by determining the point at which there is no immediately observable damage. Long-term effects or damage in conjunction with other elements can only be ascertained over time. By now we know that x-rays do some amount of damage and that exposure to them should be only when absolutely necessary.

## Concerning the Constitution Factor

Frequently I hear, "Uncle Moe smoked, drank and ate ham and potatoes and he lived to be ninety-five, so don't tell me those things are bad for me."

Well, Uncle Moe certainly proved several things. He proved that not all people are the same and he proved that he had an

*How come Uncle Moe smoked, drank and ate ham and potatoes and he lived to be ninety-five?*

exceptionally strong physical constitution. The fact is, we all do not have the same constitution and the sooner we recognize and adjust to this fact, the better.

## Concerning the Positive Factors

### Strong genes – parents both strong                    +10

*Many ancestral diseases can be avoided if we take early and consistent steps to do so.*

While this is similar to the matter of constitution, it includes an added dimension. Some regard the disease of their parents as part of their own birthright and surrender to the expectations of suffering the same. I disagree! I believe that one may inherit tendencies toward a certain disease. These, however, are not a sentence, but should put us on the alert so that we will take preventive measures. Many ancestral diseases can be avoided if we take early and consistent steps to do so. So, if you did not inherit strong genes, then eliminate a few more of the negatives in the earlier section.

### Vitamin C 1000 mg. or more daily                    +3

*Countless people experience dramatic health improvement by adding vitamin C to their daily diet.*

Vitamin C levels in the body are directly related to the body's ability to rebuild, heal and resist disease. I have seen countless people experience dramatic health improvement just by adding 1000 to 3000 mg. of vitamin C to their daily diet. Take it in 500 mg. dosages throughout the day.

### Detoxification – fasting or major detox biannually  +4

In the midst of today's polluted environment it is impossible not to become polluted internally. This toxic load carried in our bodies certainly reduces health and vitality. An ancient and still effective way to deal with this problem is fasting. See notes on this in Chapter 12. Another way that has greatly helped many thousands is a biannual bodily detoxification along with a thorough colon evacuation. I have covered this extensively in my other book, *Healthy Steps*.

### Fresh foods 70% or more of diet                         +5

Fresh foods contain live enzymes which are lost in cooking or processing. Fresh and live foods yield more live elements and a higher health potential.

*The toxic load carried in our bodies certainly reduces health and vitality.*

### Exercise – regularly 3 or more times per week          +5

Since most of us no longer hunt nor gather our food and many of us do not earn our living by physical labor, we receive inadequate exercise. The human body was made for and operates best when it frequently exerts itself physically. So, let's quit wasting time talking and writing about it. Get up and do it. You will live longer for it.

### Supplements – multi-vitamin/mineral/enzyme daily  +5

Oh yes, unless you are a brother or sister of Peter Rabbit and eat organic produce directly from the garden, supplements can make a difference. In the truest sense, supplements are simply "a concentrated additional supply" of what the body requires to maintain optimal health.

*Unless you eat organic produce directly from the garden, supplements can make a difference.*

### Basic food combining                                    +5

The combination of foods in our stomach at any given time definitely affects our digestion. This in turn influences the amount of nutrients that will be assimilated. Digestion and assimilation both have an effect on long-term health.

For more detail, see the section in Part Two on food combining.

*For details on food combining, see Chapter 9.*

Certainly other factors could be mentioned. What we have discussed is in no way exhaustive, but rather an attempt to generate awareness and activate positive behavioral changes. Consider and make your own list or add to the one above.

As these seeds of awareness are planted in daily life, they will certainly yield a harvest of a longer and healthier life.

# Chapter 6

# *Determining Your Weight Potential*

The following chapter is designed to generate an awareness of the relationship between what and how we eat, and weight control. Countless people who have a weight problem, some even very severe, seem to have little conscious awareness of why they have this problem. Meanwhile, they are dreaming of and looking for a pill or magic bullet that will solve their problem.

Occasionally I go to an "all you can eat" buffet, which I enjoy for the variety rather than for the quantity. Personally, I wish there were "half of what you can eat" buffets. Anyway, I can predict what different people will put on their plates by observing their weight. Recently, I saw a huge couple, both very obese, come in and take their seats next to ours. I asked my wife why both partners of a couple are often overweight. Her answer was "Because they both tend to eat similar food. Let's watch!"

They shuffled up to the buffet and soon returned with plates heaped with fried meats, fried potatoes and gravy, white rolls

*All of us need an awareness of the relationship between what and how we eat, and weight control.*

with loads of butter, and a little bit of fried rice. There were virtually no vegetables and nothing fresh or green. Before long this was repeated with loads of chicken – fat, skin and all. Eventually, this was followed by a humongous dish of ice cream and sugary cream tarts. Only their taste buds ended up satisfied. They left appearing tired, exhausted and heavily laden in every way, without any realization that they had just prolonged their ill health and unhappiness for another day.

*... tired, exhausted and heavily laden in every way, they had just prolonged their ill health and un-happiness for another day.*

My wife and I had an enjoyable meal with a wide variety of vegetables and tasty little snippets of fish, crab, shrimp and black beans. After slowly chewing and enjoying one plateful, I felt content and satisfied.  But, I guess I must have yielded to the atmosphere of the place when I went back for seconds – a few little tasty tidbits and even a small scoop of ice cream. So, there you have my honest confession – not really perfect but anyway it wasn't too bad and since I do it less than once a month,  my overall score and weight stays low. I hope this shows that we can enjoy food and be healthy too.

Like the age potential scale, the following is merely an attempt to link behavior and choices to real consequences. Also, rather than arguing over how much any specific food affects us, we would do well to realize the cumulative effect of similar foods. While avoiding all of the negative foods may be extreme, limiting their intake will definitely enhance one's weight control and healthy living potential.

*Limiting the intake of negative foods will definitely enhance one's weight control and healthy living potential.*

Beside each "weighty" item is a suggested "light " alternative. Generally we do not react well to being told what not to do, so be sure to also study and apply the positive suggestions found in Part 2 of this book.

### Weight Potential Scale

Column B = points per serving or incident of Column A.  C = Servings or incidents per week. D = points per week (B times C)

| A | B | C | D | Alternatives |
|---|---|---|---|---|
| Bacon, eggs and hash browns | 4 X _____ = _____ | | | grapefruit/bran muffin |
| Pie | 2 X _____ = _____ | | | fresh strawberries |
| Ice cream | 2 X _____ = _____ | | | yogurt |
| Pork, sausage, bologna | 3 X _____ = _____ | | | wholewheat bread with lettuce/tomato |
| French fries | 1 X _____ = _____ | | | roast potato wedges/carrots |
| White bread, butter, jam | 1 X _____ = _____ | | | wholewheat bread with all fruit jam |
| Potatoes w/butter | 2 X _____ = _____ | | | potato w/cottage cheese |
| Meat and gravy (over 6 oz.) | 2 X _____ = _____ | | | sm lean meat – broiled |
| Pop, 2 or more per day | 1 X _____ – _____ | | | iced herb tea/fruit juice |
| Sugary cereal | 1 X _____ = | | | hot oatmeal |
| Whole milk (more than 6 oz.) | 1 X _____ = | | | Rice or soy drink |
| Candy, choc, etc., 2+per day | 1 X _____ = _____ | | | apple, orange, pear |
| Butter, more than 2 pats per day | 1 X _____ = _____ | | | half pat butter |
| Hamburger with works | 2 X _____ = _____ | | | veggie burger |
| Second helping – except veg. | 2 X _____ = _____ | | | more vegetables |
| Dessert – after a  meal | 3 X _____ = _____ | | | herbal tea/hot water |
| Sweet snacks | 1 X _____ = _____ | | | fruit juice popsicle |
| Nibbling, except veg & fruit | 2 X _____ = _____ | | | veggies, popcorn |
| Regular salad dressing, ketchup | 1 X _____ = _____ | | | oil/vinegar dressing |
| Bedtime snacks | 2 X _____ = _____ | | | popcorn lightly buttered |
| Dinner less than 2 hrs before bedtime | 3 X _____ = _____ | | | eat earlier or snack |

*Subtotal* _____

Donuts, chips, etc.           2 X ____=____           veggies, fruit
Chicken, skin and fat         2 X ____=____           white meat, no skin

High Stress                   2 X ____=____           relax and enjoy
Toxic body                    3 X ____=____           detoxify
Days without exercise         8 X ____=____           exercise

*Total this Page* _____

*Subtotal from Previous Page* _____

**Weight Potential Total** _____

Possible excess weight relative to totals:

Over  350  60 + pounds overweight
      300 - 350  50+  pounds overweight
      250 - 300  40+
      200 - 250  30+
      150 - 200  20+
      100 - 150  10+
      under 100

Reducing your total equals reducing your weight potential!

# PART TWO

# GOOD HEALTH
# AS A DAILY PRACTICE

# Chapter 7

# Getting Clear on the Basics

In this section we get to the heart of the matter. If you miss this, you've missed it all! Regardless how much we know about our dilemma or how many natural remedies we are familiar with we will not be assured of good health. The only real assurance of good health comes from the daily, habitual practice of healthy living. On the surface, this may seem simple and it is. It may, however, be a long way from where we are now living. But, if we are willing to take small logical and manageable steps in that direction we can arrive at the goal. Even the journey can be enjoyable and the results, as illustrated from the story in the introduction, may be renewed years of health and happiness.

Living according to daily good health practice is not diffi-cult. In fact, it is natural. Breaking out of the momentum of unhealthy practices is the hard part. When we have become addicted to unhealthy living and live in an environment of health ignorance, it takes commitment and determined effort to break

*The only real assur-ance of good health comes from the daily, habitual practice of healthy*

*Part Two*
*Good Health as a Daily Practice*

free. Not to smoke is easy, once you have quit. But, for the addicted smoker who lives in a smokers' environment, breaking out of it is not automatic. Yet the effort will undoubtedly pay off with many healthy years.

As you read and determine to enter this adventure, don't be overwhelmed and don't be fanatical. Take it a little "bite" at a time. Each step will bring new satisfaction and encouragement. Don't push it, promote it or flaunt it; just quietly live it. Gradually, your shallow cravings will be replaced by deeper satisfactions and your fickle tastes will be replaced by solid appreciations.

If you "fall off the wagon," smile and get back on again. If others laugh or tease, keep smiling for they are really envying you. The social pressure you resist is far easier to deal with than the cancer, heart disease and early death they might have to fight.

Seeing my healthy eighty-eight year-old dad smiling as he worked in his own hand-tilled garden was easier than watching my seventy-seven year-old uncle die of obesity and respiratory breakdown. The choice is yours. But you have to make it early – how about now?

*Our basic premise: the human body always wants to be healthy; if it is not, it will aggressively attempt to regain its health.*

Our basic premise is and always will be: the human body always wants to be healthy, and even if it is not, it will aggressively attempt to regain its health. If we give it the care and resources it needs, it will maintain its own health for all of its years. To express this in an easily understood way, I have developed what I call the A SED theory. (Pronounced A Said.)

## The A SED Theory

This theory proposes that good health is assured if the body is Adequate in three areas: Supply, Elimination and Defense. In this chapter we will briefly explain each of these three areas. The following chapters will then develop the daily practical application of each in detail.

First of all, for the body to maintain good health the body must have an *Adequate Supply* of vital nutritional elements. If the supply is inadequate or compromised due to a lack of nutritious food, health will begin to deteriorate. If this occurs, rather than medicating to suppress the problem, we must bring in *Additional Supply* through better diet and supplementation.

**A SED Theory**

  *A* dequate

  *S* upply
  *E* limination
  *D* efense

Besides *Supply* the body must continually *Eliminate* all unused food stuff as well as body wastes and toxic accumulation. Only a clean body, free of debris and toxic waste, can maintain good health. Here again, if health suffers due to internal pollution, instead of suppressing symptoms we must *Activate* the *Elimination*. This will be the primary focus in Chapter 12 on elimination.

Bacteria, virus and fungus are constantly invading our bodies. In order to disarm the negative effects of these health robbers, we all have an amazing internal defense called the immune system. Obviously, we need *Adequate Defense* to protect us from our pollution-laden environment. In Chapter 13, we will learn how to *Assist* our *Defense* system. This is becoming more and more crucial in order to maintain good health.

Certainly all would agree that Adequate Supply, Elimination and Defense are necessary for maintaining good health. In fact, this is obviously the best form of prevention. We must now ask some questions. If this is the way to maintain health, why when health is failing would we not simply intensify this form of prevention? Why would we try to artificially attack the disease when the body has its own desire and ability to overcome the problem? Why not intensify prevention and let the body do what it can do best for itself? This is the heart of Help Yourself Health Care!

| To maintain good health<br>*Prevention* | To regain lost health<br>*Prevention Intensified* |
|---|---|
| **Adequate Supply**<br>*Proper nutrition*<br>*through food* | **Additional Supply**<br>*Supplementation*<br>*see Chapters 8 - 11* |
| **Adequate Elimination**<br>*Regularity, kidneys*<br>*and sweating* | **Activate Elimination**<br>*Detoxification*<br>*see Chapter 12* |
| **Adequate Defense**<br>*Normal immune function* | **Assist Defense**<br>*Immune support*<br>*see Chapter 13* |

Whenever someone asks me what to take for a certain disease, I ask, "How about we just get you healthy? Did you know that your body is trying to recover from your sickness? The reason it has not been successful may be due to an inadequate supply, inadequate elimination or poor immune function. If we enhance each of these areas we may see dramatic recovery. Only after we have addressed these areas is it advisable to try to directly attack the disease."

From the above we begin to see how both health and recovery are related to prevention and intensified prevention.

# Chapter 8

# *Nutrition – the Basis for Good Health*

After years of observing health and sickness, I have come to conclude that the single most important factor for good health is our eating. Behind virtually every disease or health frustration lies poor food choice. Yes, we eat loads of food, but we have become an overfed yet undernourished people. The first step to better health is not medicine or even vitamins or herbs, but proper eating. This is why, a major part of this book will be on food. If you miss this, you will receive only minimal or temporary help.

*Behind virtually every disease or health frustration lies poor food choice.*

## The Place of Nutrition in Human Health

Some years ago a young listener at one of my lectures challenged me with what he must have assumed was a rather probing question: "Sir, how long have you been into nutrition?"

I perceived that he was impressed with the thought that he had taken interest in this area earlier than most of the audience.

He seemed to want to compare himself with me. So, I responded, "I can tell you quite precisely when I first got into nutrition. It was on a cold winter day in December over one half century ago. I had just come through a major traumatic experience. Somehow, intuitively, I seemed to realize that my survival and my future health and well-being depended on my getting into nutrition. I was blessed with a most loving mother who provided me with a perfect supply, and I have been into nutrition ever since." Then I asked him, "And when did you get into nutrition?"

He grinned and muttered, "I think I get the point."

*Health begins, proceeds and ends with nutrition.*

This is the first and most basic "point" we all must "get" if we ever really want to understand health. Health begins, proceeds and ends with nutrition. Maybe we all don't need to get into the in-depth science of nutrition, but we all had better get into its daily practice. Our body is made and functions in such a way that if we practice proper nutrition, we are virtually assured of a long and healthy life. However, if we don't, either by willful refusal or by ignorance, we will pay our dues in unwanted suffering. Nutrition is this important!

While animal nutrition has been taken very seriously for years, human nutrition has been taken for granted until recently. Already in the late 1940s and early 1950s, when I was a farm boy we were very conscious about the quality of feed for the cattle. Even then, every cow received a "pinch" of mineral supplement. This supplement, which we simply called "stock food" was an additional supply of minerals. This was found to be essential for healthy and productive livestock.

Veterinarians were taught that animal health was primarily a nutritional matter. When an animal was sick, the first question asked was "What did it eat?" Since the farmer did not have animal health insurance, and "medical bills" would have made his operation unprofitable, an effective and inexpensive way had to be found to maintain animal health. That way was good nutrition including supplementation.

Read the information slip on a bag of dog chow. You will be amazed at the research and the exact nutritional balance that has gone into this feed. Pet food often is far superior in nutritional balance to the food we feed our children. This is why our pets are so much healthier than our children.

In the 1960s we purchased a beautiful American Eskimo (Spitz) dog as a family pet. Her favorite food was table scraps. Since it was cheaper than dog food, she usually got it. All leftover meat, gravy, potatoes, milk and other human goodies were hers to gorge herself on. By age 9, she began to get cancerous tumors. These were surgically removed only to have more tumors appear in far greater numbers. By age 10, she had to be put to sleep, as her body was filled with cancer.

Since we all loved this special dog, we replaced her with an identical pup. The only difference was that she was never allowed to eat anything but high quality dog food. This dog lived a super active and healthy life to age 16. The difference was so dramatic that we almost decided to live on dog food! But by then, of course, we had changed our own eating habits, and, no doubt, our table scraps would have been somewhat better.

## So, What is a Healthy Diet?

The food conscious consumer is becoming overwhelmed with a hailstorm of often conflicting directives as to what and what not to eat. Once you ask what should be a simple and sincere question, "What is good for me and my children?" be prepared to run for cover. Every self-styled expert, every "health nut" and even the ever-changing science researchers will clamor for your ear. And if that weren't enough, now the internet can bombard you with a million new "answers" from every expert and do-

*The food conscious consumer is becoming overwhelmed with a hailstorm of often conflicting directives ...*

gooder the world over who has found this new platform for spouting opinions.

So, you are dying to ask me, "Do eggs really raise cholesterol? Should we eat meat? What about milk? How much raw and how much cooked food? Is chicken okay? What about fish? How much protein do we need? What about dairy products? How do we get enough calcium? How much sugar is okay? What about salt? Are peanuts better raw or roasted? Butter or margarine? Coffee or tea? ? ? ? ? ?" Stop, stop, I hear these questions in my sleep! But, then again, perhaps if I would hear more of these questions earlier, I would hear less of the "What do I take for..." kind of questions later in people's lives.

No doubt, a big part of our problem lies in that we have conditioned people to want "yes or no" legal answers, rather than helping them to think for themselves. Of course, this state of dependency is far more profitable for the experts. However, I would much rather empower people to make their own valid decisions. You probably want specific answers on each question, and you will probably find them, even elsewhere in this book. But, I really hope you will absorb the following principles so that you can come to your own conscientious conclusions. Then, you will not be blown about every time you hear a new or different opinion, but will find and practice principles that will ensure you and your family's good health. Realizing that the basic aspects of human nutrition are food and water, we will begin by considering the matter of food. In Chapter 10 we will consider water.

*Absorb the principles so that you can come to your own conscientious conclusions.*

First, let's get clear on general principles and guidelines. Then we will look at some specifics.

Several years ago, I was honored to present a lecture along with Dr. Abram Hoffer whom I consider to be one of the world's most noble alternative health pioneers. I don't remember my lecture but I still cherish the notes I took from his. He gave us an excellent summary of good diet guidelines using six adjectives. I take the liberty to pass these on to you.

Determine as much as possible to eat foods that are:

| | | |
|---|---|---|
| Alive/recently alive | *versus* | dead |
| Whole | *versus* | processed, extracted or refined |
| Varied | *versus* | always the same, few kinds |
| Nontoxic | *versus* | additives, pollutants |
| Locally grown | *versus* | exogenous – from afar |
| Scarce | *versus* | too abundant |

A basic premise he holds is that the closer we adhere to the dietary principles our early ancestors used, the more compatible our diet will be to our bodily function and the healthier we will be.

I will now present my own personal list with interpretations based on my research and experience.

## Principles For Healthy Eating

*1. Eat whole, fresh, unrefined and unprocessed foods, as soon after harvesting and as close to their natural state as possible – organically grown preferred.*

Such foods will supply the delicate vitamins, necessary enzymes and essential fatty acids which we often lack. They will also assure us adequate fiber which is lost in refining and processing, and reduce the toxic load from additives, preservatives, flavorings and colorings.

*whole, fresh, unrefined and unprocessed foods*

*2. Eat a wide variety of different vegetables, fruits, grains and nuts.*

Try not to eat the same food every day. Do not eat excessive amounts of any one food. Generally less is better than more!

Since no one food contains all essential elements, a broad variety will greatly limit the possibility of certain deficiencies. This will also greatly reduce the possibility of developing food

*wide variety of different foods*

*Many people dig their graves with their dinner forks.*

allergies. Research has shown that animals fed less than they would choose to eat far outlive those that overindulge. A wise sage once said, "Many people dig their graves with their dinner forks."

*3. Eat primarily the natural foods that were healthy for your ancestors.*

*Eat foods healthy for your ancestors.*

For example, Northern European people historically ate meat and dairy, so generally their descendants can digest and assimilate these foods more easily. Africans and Asians traditionally did not consume dairy products and their descendants are much more prone to lactose intolerance and dairy allergies. Rather than accepting and trying to apply a blanket eat or don't eat this or that, consider the diet of your ancestors and factor that into your food choices.

*4. Learn and practice the basic principles of proper food combining.*

*For more details on food combining, see Chapter 9.*

Good digestion and maximum absorption of nutrients in food is greatly enhanced by applying the principles of basic food combining. Since effective digestion of fruit and protein require a very different process, it should be obvious that these are best eaten separately.

*5. Moderate your eating depending on your level of activity and biochemistry.*

*Adjust eating relative to activity levels.*

Too often we forget to adjust our eating relative to our activity levels. Many very physically active farmers consume great quantities of fat, meat and dairy yet they remain reasonably healthy. However, soon after they retire and become inactive, their health breaks down and most are outlived by their wives.

I still see this phenomena when I visit retired relatives in an area of Florida popular with retired farmers. Often the most strenuous activity among some of these people is what someone called "having a good brisk sit." The restaurants still cater to these farm folks' traditional appetites and prepare mountains of meat and buttered mashed potatoes to be flooded with gravy and followed with lavish deserts. I have commented that these restaurants should have a slogan like "Welcome, come in and eat yourself to death."

*Exercise more or eat less!*

If these men would alter their eating habits to match their lifestyle change, many would be healthier and might significantly extend their lifetime. Their wives never had the habit of eating as heavily and now after retirement tend to remain more physically active. (Women do seem to be genetically programed to live longer as well.) So, of course, most of them outlive their husbands.

If we would understand and apply these five basic principles, many of the confusing questions would be resolved. For example, if you follow these principles, the questions about how much fat, cholesterol or sugar will be already resolved. It will also be apparent that not everyone has to eat the same thing. For example, if you are chopping wood, digging ditches or climbing ladders eight to ten hours a day, you can afford to eat large and hardy meals. If your most vigorous activity is "running up" your charge account, and "jumping" to conclusions, then you had best eat much less, with only very small amounts of fat and animal products. Realistically speaking we know, of course, that the reader will still have some specific questions and we will attempt to address them as we proceed.

## Before We Eat – Time for a Healthy Pause

Have you considered lately the beauty and wonder of food? It is an amazing phenomena that the life of plants can be used to convey life and energy to us so that we can continue living. The continuation of our life is absolutely dependent on food. We could live without most everything we think we need, but not without food. Isn't food an indispensable and wonderful gift that we take too much for granted?

Real food cannot be made by man, it must be grown. What makes it grow? Where does the color in the carrot and the beet come from? Who can extract the taste of the onion or the radish from soil? How can that same soil produce hot peppers and sweet corn? Food really is a miracle and not merely the result of man's ingenuity. Furthermore, it grows without charge! All the money you pay for it goes to the people who cultivated or handled it, not one penny went to the One who caused it to grow, or who first created the life in the initial seed! How could anyone not be inspired to give thanks?

## Beginning With a Thankful Heart

I believe that an important part of total health and happiness includes being thankful, an attitude which we all might do well to cultivate.

In my childhood home we always gave thanks or "said grace" before we ate. As children, we saw it mostly as a delay to getting at the good food mom had prepared. So, we became experts at making our "grace" as short as possible. The shortest prayer we were able to get away with was "Thank the Lord, Amen!"

*If it is good courtesy to thank the cook, how about thanking the Creator?*

I remember one time as a child asking an uncle why the chickens raised their heads and made a gurgling sound every time they took a swallow of water. "They are giving thanks," he replied.

I'm not sure how scientific his answer was, but it made an impression on me, and "giving thanks" has remained a part of our family and my personal mealtime enjoyment. It has become much more special to me since I now have a personal relationship with the provider of my food.

We've paid the persons who have cultivated or prepared it, and we've thanked the cook. Whatever or Whoever it is that made it grow hasn't asked for pay or anything, so, isn't it appropriate for us to be thankful to what or Whoever we believe that is? Besides, a thankful heart makes us happier and more content, and that is even good for digestion.

*A thankful heart makes us happier and more content, and that is even good for digestion.*

# Chapter 9

# Food Specifics –
# What? Why? and How?

We are constantly bombarded with often contradictory advice on what we should eat. Almost every month some new diet is put forward. Unfortunately, these diets are often so detailed and restrictive, that they are almost impossible to follow. Furthermore, they only work for a small percentage of the select few who are able to stick to them. People are becoming discouraged and overwhelmed as they seek to escape this dietary confusion.

Once we are clear on the basic principles of nutrition as outlined in the previous chapter, it is time to look at some specific guidelines. While these guidelines must be detailed enough to be easily applicable, they must also be simple enough to be workable for everyone. I trust that what I lay before you in this chapter will serve to clarify the current dietary dilemma.

*People are becoming discouraged and overwhelmed as they seek to escape this dietary confusion.*

## To Cook or Not to Cook

Should we cook our food, how much and with what?

*Fruit*

Fruit is almost always best for us when eaten raw, preferably fresh or if frozen, eaten immediately after being thawed. Canned fruit has comparatively little value as many of the vitamins and virtually all of the natural enzymes have been destroyed. Fruit is very easily and quickly digested and is best if eaten by itself. The worst time to eat fruit is after a meal. Most people who conclude that fruit does not agree with them have a problem because they eat it with starch and protein. (See more on this under food combining.) Eat fruit by itself and discover how healthful and invigorating it is. "An apple a day keeps the doctor away" was not an unwise truism.

*Vegetables*

Eat raw vegetables in salads or as veggie sticks. A preferred dressing is flax seed oil, grape seed oil or olive oil. Some would argue that all foods should be eaten raw. I believe this is an extreme view. Although it may be a great short-term therapy, and some people may do well on it over the long-term, it is not for everyone. (For a well-balanced view on this refer to Paul and Patricia Bragg's book, *Healthful Eating Without Confusion*, pages 41-42.)

*Grape seed and flax seed oils should not be heated.*

When cooking vegetables, steam them or try a quick stir-fry using extra virgin olive oil, or canola oil. When vegetables are cooked until they are soft, their real food value is mostly lost. Incidentally, some of what is lost is in the juice, so don't throw that away; use it! The taste is also lost, and this is why the consumer automatically dumps loads of salt on to try to revive some taste in the deadened food.

To steam or stir-fry, use stainless steel pots; do not use aluminium. Some of the aluminium will inevitably leach out and will contaminate the food. If you use Teflon, be very sure that the coating is not scratched or marred. Leakage from the coating may be toxic, and any damaged pan should not be used for food.

Meat should be boiled, roasted, broiled, baked, stir-fried or grilled. Pork, which I certainly do not recommend for human diet, should be well done in order to destroy parasites which are very common. Beef, chicken and turkey should be at least medium well done, so that they are thoroughly heated. Fish requires less cooking time.

*Meat*

The standard programed nutritionists have been taught and assume that microwave cooking is even preferable, because the food is exposed to heat for a shorter time. I must admit that I have found little definite evidence to the contrary. So, do I have any basis at all for my "hunches" about this matter?

*Microwave cooking*

I have always had a deep reservation about microwave cooking. How can the food molecules be activated to the point of generating heat without severe damage occurring to the life elements? How can these waves be so dangerous and harmful to our body yet perfectly safe for our food?

I have seen a report that infant care nurses have been advised not to heat breast milk in the microwave for small infants as it may damage the nutritional content. Apparently babies do not do well on it. We also know two senior couples who decided to do all of their food preparation in a microwave. Within several years both of the men suffered prostate cancer. Maybe a coincidence? Maybe not.

In the meantime, we use a microwave only on rare occasions! It may be just one more of those small assaults on our health which we don't need. I would certainly rather be safe than sorry!

## What To Eat – Meat? Dairy? Eggs?

To consume the above three food groups or not to consume them is the subject of endless debate with entire books written on the merits and demerits of each. I will not present all the arguments. If you wish to get into all the details, go to the library, but be prepared – you may get overwhelmed and confused. I will simply offer my own observations. Since I have no interests in either a dairy, egg farm or vegetable growers union, I hope I can be somewhat objective. I will expand on this matter under the topic of vegetarianism.

*Meat*

As a general rule I have to conclude that most North Americans would be healthier if they ate much less meat than they do. I would rate meat in general, from least preferable to most preferable, as follows: processed meats, pork, beef, lamb, chicken, turkey, rabbit, fish, wild game. Meat should only be eaten as a special food. Take small bites, chew well, savor and enjoy it, but only a maximum of two to six ounces per meal, and never more than once per day. If you use meat as the main part of your meal, then I can "bet you a whole cow" that you have digestion problems and will not remain healthy and active in your older years. If your physical activity is equal to the amount that it would require to hunt and prepare the wild game, then you might constructively utilize a larger portion.

Personally, I do not eat pork, including bacon. I eat only small amounts of beef perhaps once a week. Several days per week, I eat no meat. I feel that with this arrangement, my body performs best, much better than when I ate large amounts of meat twice daily and also better then when I tried vegetarianism. I urge you to be honest and listen to your body rather than your appetite in order to find the healthy amount of meat for you.

*Tips for eating meat.*

If you wish to use hamburger, have it ground just before you eat it and cook it well. The growth potential of bacteria is greatly accelerated in ground meat. Remove as much fat as possible, take the skin off chicken, pour away the grease and let it plug the sink drains instead of your arteries. At the same time be aware that the body needs certain fats in order to be healthy. These fats are known as essential fatty acids and are very important. So, don't go on a no-fat kick and fall off the other side of the wagon. See more on fats later.

Welcome to another topic that has been kicked about, churned with controversy and fermented with much propaganda. Let me give a summary of my conclusions with a brief explanation for each.

**Dairy Products**

*Cow's milk is natures's perfect food only if you are a baby cow!* The nutritional profile of cow's milk and human milk is quite different. For instance, cow's milk contains 21 percent protein whereas human milk contains only 5 percent protein. Cow's milk is certainly not an ideal substitute for breast milk and can never provide an infant with adequate nutrition in the early formative months. If introduced early in life, it will often instigate lactose intolerance.

*The health of many children and some adults is significantly frustrated because they have unknown milk allergies or lactose intolerance.* Studies cited by John Robbins in *May All Be Fed* found that 90 percent of Filipinos and Japanese, 70 percent of African Americans, 65 percent of Mexican Americans, 50 percent of Indians, and over 10 percent of Caucasians are lactose intolerant. Personally, among the Caucasians I deal with, I find a rate much higher than 10 percent. I believe that the homogenization process which breaks up the fat molecules into smaller than normal fragments may be a reason. These molecules may pass through the gut wall undigested and can provoke the immune system into an allergic response. I have seen many sickly children with stuffy heads, runny noses, dark-circled eyes, skin rashes, earaches and listlessness recover quickly when taken off dairy products.

*Milk is not necessary in order to get adequate calcium.* Countries where dairy consumption is highest also have the highest rate of calcium deficiency diseases. Millions of children in this world never drink milk and never suffer from calcium deficiency.

In fact, the highest incidence of osteoporosis is found in the countries where dairy consumption is highest (Sweden, U.S., Finland and the United Kingdom). The incidence of osteoporosis is lowest where the least amount of dairy products is consumed (Asian and African countries).

*Calcium is in all foods that grow from the soil; humans can get it just as easily as the cows can.*

Calcium is found in all foods that grow from the soil and humans can get it from there just as easily as the cows can. The cows do not need to drink milk or eat meat to get calcium and neither do we. Also, be aware that in order for calcium to be transported into the body tissue, it must be accompanied by magnesium, very little of which is found in cow's milk.

*Milk that has been pasteurized, homogenized and fortified, and comes from cows which have been vaccinated and fed chemicals is no longer a pure natural food.* Raw certified, non-homogenized milk is preferable but rarely available.

*Butter versus margarine*

*Butter is better than margarine, but eat it sparingly.* During World War II while Europe had its supply of margarines and shortening cut off, it witnessed the steepest decline in heart disease in this century. After the war when margarine was again available, heart disease rates increased again!

*Many conditions, such as MS, respiratory illness, ulcers, bowel problems, nasal congestion, headaches, eczema and hives, etc. are often relieved when dairy products are discontinued.*

John Robbins states, "The list of the most common symptoms of dairy allergies is a long one, as are the benefits often obtained by allergic people who remove dairy products from their diet. Many studies have shown allergies to dairy products to cause irritability, restlessness, hyperactivity, muscle pain, mental depression, abdominal pain, cramps or bloating, gas, diarrhea, bad breath, headaches, lack of energy, constipation, poor appetite, poor absorption of nutrients, nasal stuffiness, runny nose, sinusitis, asthma, shortness of breath, rashes, eczema and hives."

It is easy to see if one is allergic to dairy products. For five days avoid all forms of dairy intake, including butter, cheese, ice cream and milk, even in coffee. On the sixth day, drink several ounces of milk. Observe your body's reactions both during the time of abstinence and upon resuming intake. If each day of the five saw general health improvement and day six evoked significant negative reactions, then the answer is clear; your body's immune system has determined that dairy products are an enemy and must be fought against. This battle exhausts the immune system so that it cannot maintain overall health. In this case, dairy products should be avoided.

*Test for dairy allergy*

If there is no observable difference in health after dairy products are reintroduced, this indicates that they are not a problem and may be taken without negative effects.

*Some people, but very few blacks and Asians, can tolerate and even receive some health benefits from milk.*

If your ancestors have been milk drinkers, you may be able to benefit from it and enjoy it. I am not for or against milk; I am for good health! I trust that the above can help you rise above the advertising hype and make a healthy informed decision on the matter.

The matter of whether to eat eggs is about as delicate as walking on egg shells. John Robbins, a conscientious nutritionist but avowed vegetarian, seems to prove that they raise cholesterol and do not belong in the human diet. Paul Bragg, an honored life extension specialist, sees them as a nutritious form of food if eaten in moderation. Robert Crayhon, a respected nutrition researcher, insists that they do not raise cholesterol. So, what should we do? Close our eyes and eat them, or rebuke them as evil.

*Eggs*

I have to conclude that eggs can be a significant form of food if eaten fresh, in moderation, along with other food and not daily. Two eggs a day with bacon, toast and hash browns probably significantly increase cholesterol and pose a hazardous health risk. I certainly appreciate a free-range farm fresh egg on occasion, perhaps once or twice a week. I no longer enjoy the factory eggs laid by force-fed chickens confined in a two foot square prison, under artificial light and without exercise. Without exercise the cholesterol which the hen would burn up running around and the toxins that she would excrete are passed on in the egg – how can such an egg be healthy?

Give me a fresh, fertile, deeply orange-yolked egg that stands up and smiles at me and I won't resist. For that I will make an "eggception!"

## How Much? – Protein, Sugar, Fats

*Protein*

High protein, low protein, animal protein, protein first, last or alone – every day there's a new theory and every week a new book. Where's the beef on this matter?

First, let's consider how much protein a human needs for maintenance of good health. Somehow, we have come to believe that we need lots of protein and that the more we can get, the better for us. Even small children are indoctrinated to believe that they must eat lots of protein if they want to become big and strong.

The World Health Organization, the Food and Nutrition Board of the National Academy of Sciences, and the National Research Council say that, at the very most, we need only eight percent of our daily total calories from protein. Human breast milk contains five percent of its calories from protein. Furthermore, the average American consumes 90 to 120 grams of protein per day, whereas the ideal intake for human beings is only 30 to 50 grams per day. While many are worrying about not getting enough protein, most are eating far more than necessary and even more than is healthy.

Before the body can use protein for energy it must convert

it into glucose. This is done in the liver and requires a high amount of metabolic energy. This is why a high protein diet often leaves one quite exhausted. No wonder the big meat eater needs a rest after eating! Even lions need to rest after eating meat.

Many athletes have bought into the more protein is better myth and are consuming far too much. Excess protein can stress the kidneys and liver, and drain calcium from the bone stores. While lean muscle tissue does require more protein, even the most active athlete needs little more than 100 grams per day.

Harvey and Marilyn Diamond in *Living Health* (page 241) document conclusively that excess protein severely inhibits the body's absorption of calcium. The more protein (animal and dairy products) consumed, the more calcium is lost. Consequently, the number one cause of osteoporosis is consumption of animal products. Yet many eat the dairy products to get more calcium.

There are many foods other than animal products that contain significant amounts of protein. The chart on the following page shows conclusively that animal products are not the only source of protein.

Another excellent source is spirulina which is 70 percent protein, and is no doubt the best non-animal protein source.

In 1971, Frances Moore Lappe published a book entitled *Diet for a Small Planet.* She declared that if people properly combined vegetable proteins they would get all the amino acids necessary, and not need to eat animal products. This seemed to be good news for vegetarians but still left some concern about proper combinations.

After further research, Lappe wrote a revised edition in 1982. In this book she states that since her first edition she has found that to get enough protein without meat is much easier than she had earlier thought. She concluded that with a healthy varied diet, concern about protein complementariness is not necessary,

*A healthy varied diet: wide selection of vegetables, whole grains, legumes, nuts, seeds and fruit.*

## Percentage of Calories from Protein

### Grains

| | | | |
|---|---|---|---|
| broccoli | 36% | soybean curd | 40% |
| brussels sprouts | 36% | soybeans | 32% |
| cabbage | 18% | split peas | 28% |
| carrots | 10% | white beans | 26% |
| cauliflower | 10% | | |

### Nuts and seeds

| | | | |
|---|---|---|---|
| cucumbers | 20% | almonds | 11% |
| kale | 40% | cashews | 12% |
| lettuce | 29% | peanuts | 18% |
| green peas | 30% | pumpkin seeds | 20% |
| bell peppers | 20% | sunflower seeds | 17% |
| potatoes | 11% | walnuts | 13%. |
| spinach | 40% | | |
| tomatoes | 17% | | |
| watercress | 40% | | |
| zucchini | 26% | | |

**Fruits** provide relatively small amounts of protein ranging from apples at 1% to cherries, cantaloupes, grapes, oranges, raspberries and strawberries all at 8%.

### Grains

| | |
|---|---|
| barley | 9% |
| buckwheat | 13% |
| oatmeal | 15% |
| brown rice | 8% |
| dark rye flour | 18% |
| spaghetti | 14% |
| whole wheat | 16% |
| wheat germ | 29% |

**For comparison** most cheese ranges in the 23% range, except cottage cheese at 52%.

| | |
|---|---|
| whole eggs | 33% |
| milk | 21% |
| low fat yogurt | 27% |
| lean beef | 32% |
| chicken, dark meat | 67% |
| chicken, white meat | 81% |
| lamb | 32% |
| perch | 33% |
| pork | 23% |
| turkey | 41% |

**Legumes** – excellent as a source of protein, all are above 20%, some of the highest are:

| | |
|---|---|
| broad beans | 31% |
| cowpeas | 28% |
| kidney beans | 26% |
| lima beans | 29% |

These figures are from Nutritive value of American Foods in Common Units, Agriculture Handbook No 456.

and if people are getting enough calories, they are virtually certain of getting enough protein.

One of the greatest frustrations to the human body is refined sugar. Our digestive system and metabolism are made to process and utilize natural sugars known as complex carbohydrates found in fruit and other whole foods. These supply nutrients and energy for bodily function. If perchance the sugar level in the blood gets too high, the pancreas produces insulin and brings the sugar level down. This is an emergency protective measure and was never intended as a routine experience.

*Sugar*

When refined sugar is introduced into the body, not only is it void of any nutrients, but worse, it places a tremendous stress on the body's metabolism, setting it into a state of emergency. While the system temporarily may be able to cope, it was never made to handle this abnormal shock on a regular basis.

*Refined sugar has no vitamins or minerals. To digest it, the body must pull nutrients from its stores, leaving you quickly feeling weak and fatigued. As little as two teaspoons disrupts the balance in blood chemistry.*

Americans eat an average of 133 pounds of sugar per year. There is no doubt that this is one of the major causes of the rise in heart disease, adult onset diabetes, immune dysfunction and premature aging.

Sugar consumption has been shown:

- to cause heart disease, varicose veins and gallstones;
- to damage the kidneys;
- to cause and worsen arthritis and migraines;
- to increase the risk of breast cancer;
- to increase cholesterol, triglycerides and insulin levels;
- to deplete B vitamins and chromium, and interfere with the absorption of calcium and magnesium;
- to weaken the immune system;
- to increase the acidity of the stomach; and
- to contribute to obesity.

All of the above effects have been documented. Knowing the damaging effects of sugar, why would any rational, intelligent person indulge in such a deadly substance?

It must be because it also apparently overrules the willpower of otherwise sane and normal people. To overcome this insidious destroyer of our health requires a deliberate training of our appetites and taste and an active healthy dose of willpower! But the price is small compared to the greater health and longer and better quality of life.

Some believe that since they no longer eat sugar directly, but now use honey, maple syrup and rice syrup; they have dealt with this issue. While these are preferable, they are still very intense and highly concentrated. It takes thirty gallons of maple sap to produce one gallon of syrup, and hundreds of "beeloads" per teaspoon of honey. Even these should be used only rarely, perhaps a few times a week as a treat, and only if your health is good.

Many school children's health is compromised and their learning capacity is frustrated by the sugar loaded snacks. Give your kids a real health break and get them off sugar.

Many readers were probably anticipating that I would be down on fats. Surprise! Not all fat is bad! There are two kinds of fat: nonessential fats, the bad ones, and essential fats, the good ones. Guess which ones we get too much of and which we get too little of. In fact, cutting down on fats gets some people into trouble, because when we are short in essential fats our body suffers.

*Fats*

Among the fats we consume, two fatty acids are essential: linoleic acid, also known as omega-6, and linolenic, known as omega-3. These cannot be synthesized by the body; they must come from our diet. Flax seed is the best available source of both omega-6 and omega-3. These essential fatty acids are sometimes referred to as vitamin F, and are available in supplemental form from evening primrose oil, borage oil, black currant seed oil, and flax seed oil.

*Essential Fats*

Linoleic acid, omega-6, is the most prevalent and is found in raw seeds, nuts, whole grains, corn, safflowers, sunflowers, soybeans, and avocados. When these are processed into various man-made oils, much of the linoleic acid is destroyed. Frying or other exposure to heat, light or air also breaks down linoleic acid and may produce free radicals which are also found in rancid oils.

Linolenic acid is important to reduce cholesterol, to relieve angina pectoris, bring down high blood pressure, and to help arthritis, psoriasis and eczema. It is less easily available, but is found in flax seed, fresh walnuts, chia seeds, pumpkins, and soy and canola oils.

It has been recently discovered that the Omega-3 fats are necessary for the complete development of the human brain during pregnancy and early life. Infant formula is short of this oil and even breast milk can be deficient if the mother's supply of Omega-3 is limited. One researcher found that families who had "flax" babies ended up with bright healthy children with fewer health problems than most young children experience.

*"Flax" babies ended up bright and healthy with fewer health problems.*

Fats are either saturated or unsaturated, in other words either solid or liquid. Saturated fats are best avoided. Some oils are solidified by being hydrogenated to make margarines and shortening and are found in cereals, snacks, candies, cakes and breads. Hydrogenated oils do much of the damage attributed to fats and must be avoided.

The healthy oils are flax seed oil and grape seed oil which should not be heated, canola oil, extra virgin olive oil and peanut oil, which are best for heating as in stir-frys.

(For the percentages of fat in foods, see protein/fats chart in Robbins' *May All Be Fed,* page 385.)

## Food Combining

Some healthy eating advocates make food combining very complicated. Don't eat protein with carbohydrates. Don't mix this with that. The fact is that many of the "do not mix" factors are often found in one particular plant. Legally adhering to strict guidelines can be totally impractical and not in harmony with nature.

Proper food combining does, however, have some validity. There is good reason to allow a meal of vegetables, meat and grains to digest for at least one hour before eating refined carbohydrates. This makes our North American habit of after dinner an unhealthy custom. (Someone has noted that desserts spelled backwards equals stressed.)

When the main course of a meal has been eaten, it requires several hours for complete digestion. The refined carbohydrates in desserts require very little time. If they are dumped on top of a protein, fat and complex carbohydrate meal, the digestive process is greatly frustrated. The usual result is fermentation which produces gas, indigestion and poor use of food nutrients.

*Desserts spelled backwards equals stressed, especially after meals.*

### Basic Food Combining Principles

Strictly adhering to the following principles may seem idealistic and perhaps unrealistic. However, the closer we follow them, the easier it will be for our digestive system. Applying the principles more strictly may speed recovery from health challenges. Since there is some valid basis for proper food combining let's consider the basic tenants.

Refined carbohydrates. e.g. sweets – best avoided; if eaten, take small amounts by themselves.

Fruits – best eaten by themselves, not along with or after a meal; allow at least two hours after a full meal.

Protein – e.g. meat, dairy, etc. – okay if eaten with vegetables, not with starches.

Starches – e.g. rice, potatoes – okay if eaten with vegetables, not with protein.

The primary reason for the above principles lies in the fact that different digestive enzymes are required for the best digestion of various food elements. For example, fruit requires almost no digestion, whereas protein requires high amounts of pancreatin and other enzymes, and takes several hours for complete digestion. When fruit eaten with protein remains in the stomach for very long, it begins to ferment and produce gas and indigestion. This is why some people believe that fruit does not agree with them.

Whoever started the idea of having fruit as a dessert after a meal has wrought endless devastation to digestion and generated much health frustration. Yet, we all fall in line like hapless sheep led to the slaughter. We feel great after a meal. Then we have dessert and feel stuffed and bloated, but it never dawns on us that we are choosing habit over health.

## The Body's Three Phases

The Diamonds, in their classic book, *Fit for Life*, put forward some very worthy principles. They believe that the body passes through three phases in each twenty-four hour cycle: ingestion, made up primarily of eating, normally takes place from about noon to eight in the evening; assimilation, the time for absorbing nutrients, takes place from eight in the evening until four in the morning; and elimination, the third phase, takes place preferably from four in the morning until noon.

*Ingestion*
*Assimilation*
*Elimination*

The body functions best when these cycles are respected and the body is allowed to concentrate exclusively on each phase. This means that it is advisable not to eat in the morning until noon. In this way the body can concentrate on proper and adequate elimination. Of course, this flies in the face of conventional eating habits. What about the need for energy from a good breakfast you ask? The common American breakfast requires as much energy to digest as it provides, and in the meantime it frustrates the body's elimination cycle.

If you insist that you must eat before noon, then eat only fresh fruit. Why? Because fruit when it is eaten by itself requires very minimal digestion and so interferes as little as possible with the elimination cycle.

I generally adhere to the above principles and find that the practice bears its own proof. Eating a fruit breakfast, sometimes with some granola or yogurt, makes me feel lighter and more energetic than the old-fashioned eggs, etc. breakfast. Don't knock it; try it for a month and let the results speak for themselves.

# Chapter 10

# *More Water Please*

The most abundant and most necessary element for all life is water. It is also the most crucial factor in maintaining human health. At birth the human body is over 90 percent water. By age three, the average body hydration is 75 percent, and adult levels dip as low as 65 percent. Below 60 percent death occurs. Water is crucial for health and vitality. No wonder so many people feel like a wrung-out wash rag and look like a solar-dried prune.

## Water as a Solvent

Water is necessary to carry nutrients and energy into every cell of the body. All food substance must be liquefied before they are available to body cells. Water also carries toxicity and waste products out of the cells. How can it be an effective cleansing agent if it is polluted itself? I am convinced that pure clean water, and lots of it, is an absolute necessity for excellent health.

*Water carries nutrients and energy into every cell and toxicity and waste products out of the cells.*

When in her fifties, my wife's mother was facing many health frustrations. Among the measures she employed in order to regain her health was drinking more water. She became convinced that she needed to drink much more water. So, she now fills two quarts of water every morning. One must be gone by noon and the second one by bedtime. Today, she is 80 and is an active, out-every-day, on-the-go senior. Her doctor told her some time ago, "If all my patients drank as much water as you do, I would have only half as much business as I do now."

*"If all my patients drank more water, I'd have only half as much business as I do now."*
                    *medical doctor*

## Water May Be the Most Inexpensive Cure For Many Diseases!

In a recent book *Your Body's Many Cries For Water*, Dr. F. Batmanghelidji contends that in our advanced cultures we are conditioned to ignore thirst signals. His studies conclude that chronic dehydration is at the root of conditions such as arthritis, allergies, chronic fatigue, asthma, angina, and hypertension. In fact Dr. Batmanghelidji successfully cures diseases such as asthma simply by having the patients drink great amounts of water.

We often misinterpret our body's cry for water and try to satisfy ourselves with more food. In order to cater to our whims and tastes, we substitute water with coffee, tea, soda pop and alcoholic beverages. Since these water substitutes put a stress on our bodies and must first be filtered and purified by our bodies, they can never be effective for the body's own cleansing. I believe that here lies one of the most common reasons for poor health among children. Many children drink very little water. Often they drink only pop and sweetened, artificially flavored drinks. This puts a load on the immune system and pollutes rather than cleanses their kidneys.

*Water substitutes stress our bodies, and must be filtered and purified by our bodies*

## Water Purification

No doubt, a major reason we do not drink more water is that our bodies have a subtle distaste for the polluted water we provide, calling only for a minimal amount. I can only conclude that those who wish to take natural good health seriously must take steps to purify their water supply. I have sold and used various water treatment products for many years. Presently, I do not sell such products, so I trust that I can be reasonably objective in giving the following advice.

*Those who take good health seriously must take steps to purify their water supply.*

The simplest, easiest, and very least one can do is to use filtration, such as carbon with silver. This is reasonably effective, but is limited in that it collects and holds the pollutants and loses its effectiveness with use. Carbon, by itself, can easily become a breeding ground for bacteria and should probably be changed even more frequently than suggested by the manufacturers. Although limited in its value, filtration is better than nothing.

More effective than basic filtration is reverse osmosis (RO). This should be a three stage system with pre-filter, RO module, and carbon post-filter. The pre and post-filters should be changed at least annually, and the RO module must be flushed regularly.

Ozonation, which is used to increase the oxygenation level of the water may be a preferred choice for those who are in therapeutic situations. It seems a little excessive for general use.

*water purification methods*

Ultra violet light has some value but is mostly effective for killing bacteria or other live elements, and of itself offers little benefit in cleaning up chemicals in the water.

The most effective water purification is distillation. There are presently user-friendly, compact units which overcome the inconvenience and high maintenance needs of older units. The distilled water should pass through a final carbon filter. Since distillation removes all of the trace minerals, it is advisable to add some to the water before consumption. This will also overcome the flat taste peculiar to distilled water. Two to four drops of concentrated sea source trace minerals per liter are excellent for this purpose.

There are books written on each of the above systems, each putting forward their method as the ultimate answer. I have heard, read and tested extensively in this matter and the above, without citing all the arguments, are simply my present conclusions. If you want to know the strengths of any system, ask a salesman. If you want to know the weaknesses, ask the competition.

Although bottled water is preferable to tap water, control and testing are very general, so quality can vary greatly. Spring and mountain water are mostly hype. Take responsibility, and clean your own.

## When To Drink Water

Upon rising, rinse your mouth with clean room temperature water. Drink a cup of warm water as soon as possible. These two steps will flush the toxicity accumulated through the night. This is what I call taking an internal bath and is actually more important for good health than taking an external one.

Many people get up, take a shower and have a cup of coffee. This is to begin the day by cleansing the outside and polluting the inside of your body. In order to get the impact of what you are doing, why not pour the coffee over your body and see how clean you will be!

*Taking an internal bath is actually more important than taking an external one.*

Incidentally, we have become so obsessed with external cleaning. Only under rare conditions do we need to bathe or shower more than once a day; often every other day is sufficient. Some skin specialists believe that some skin problems are related to many baths and too much soap.

Drink sparkling clean water regularly throughout the day. Don't wait until mealtime to drink all of your water. A cup of hot water with dinner is fine. It can aid digestion and help to moisten the food. A large amount of ice water is a drag on the digestive system. It chills the stomach, hardens the fats and over dilutes the digestive juices. According to the *Annals of Internal Medicine* (96:614), ice water, when passing through the esophagus next to the heart, can induce serious abnormalities of the heart rhythm for persons who have an enlarged heart.

*A large amount of ice water is a drag on the digestive system.*

Many older persons hesitate to drink water late in the day because they do not wish to arise at night. This is a mistake, and may be one reason why they have poor health. They are trading a little bit of convenience for a toxic body. Since the toxins are not regularly flushed out of the body, they overpower the immune system, and the person is susceptible to infection, virus, flu, colds and general sluggishness. To the older and to all, I say drink much, drink often, and "go" often. Whenever we refuse the urge to eliminate, we are forcing our bodies to accumulate toxicity. This is one reason why truck drivers become unhealthy. They "tank up" with coffee and "hold it" because it's not convenient to stop very often. However you work it out, do your health a favor and "go when you gotta go!"

Recently I was contacted on behalf of a woman who was greatly overweight and had a serious water retention problem. I suggested that she drink much more water. She said she could not do that because she was already retaining too much fluid. I explained that the body needs to hold fluid and fat cells in an attempt to safely store the accumulated toxins which it is unable to flush out of the system. By simply drinking much more water she improved dramatically.

Amazingly, water is not only able to help maintain health, in many cases it may be the key to regaining lost health.

# Chapter 11

# A Summary of Healthy Elements and a Place for Supplementation

Let me begin with my definition of supplements, just so we are talking the same language:

*Supplements are highly concentrated forms of vital nutrients which the human body needs and is able to utilize to maintain health and vitality.*

Is there a real need for supplements, or is this just a ploy to dupe consumers into paying good money merely to enrich the sewers of our cities? Dietitians, the primary group of traditionally trained nutritionists, are taught and declare that supplementation is unnecessary. Cardiologists generally do not recommend supplements to their patients. Yet, according to Bruce Jancin in *Family Practice News* March 1, 1994, two-thirds of these dietitians personally take supplements, and two-thirds of cardiologists take supplements to protect their own arteries and hearts.

The U.S. Surgeon General reported that he believes that 68 percent of all deaths in the United States are related to diet. So

*Two-thirds of dietitians and cardiologists take supplements.*

why the big controversy? If there is any possibility that supplements might be helpful, why not recommend them.

I have no doubt in my mind that there is much more at stake than what meets the eye. To acknowledge the value and recommend the use of supplements would be a tremendous threat to the existing medical monopoly of the health industry. If and when the medical profession can have full control of supplements, their use will be encouraged and they will be prescribed freely.

In the meantime, health care consumers are intimidated and kept dependent on the system with subtle warnings about the possible danger of taking supplements. The best answer to this scare tactic is to look at the facts.

*Deaths in America in 1992: 125,000 from prescription drugs, 9,000 from food poisoning, 0 from supplements.*

*– Why the panic?*

According to the National Center for Health Statistics, 1992 saw 125,000 people in America die as a result of taking prescription drugs, and 9,000 more die from food poisoning. That same year not one person died due to the use of vitamin and mineral supplements! If there is any possibility at all that supplements might help recover health, would not even cold, logical statistics argue that they should be recommended before drugs? After all, they appear to be even safer than food!

Personally, in my nearly twenty years of direct health involvement with thousands of people, I have seen many who have taken mega doses of vitamins. A good number have taken far greater amounts than I would recommend, yet I have never seen even one case where significant harm has been done. Yes, excess supplementation can be wasteful, but no more dangerous or harmful then excess food.

*You do not need to take supplements if...*

In response to the question, "Is there anyone who does not need supplements?" I have put forward the following answer.

You do not need to take supplements if:
– The food you eat is organically grown in mineral and nutrient rich soil.

- The food you eat was mature and ripened on the vines, plants or trees.
- The food is consumed within a few days of harvesting.
- You eat a wide variety of foods, mostly fresh and raw.
- You do not eat processed, deep fried junk food or candy.
- You drink at least 2 liters or 8 cups of pure water daily.
- You are not being exposed to chemicals in food, air or water.
- You have only occasional stress.
- You get adequate rest in clean fresh air.
- You are not exposed to electromagnetic emissions from appliances, TV, etc.
- Your body is not exposed to mercury, lead, aluminium or other heavy metals.
- You fast or detoxify your body and colon at least twice a year.

I'll be honest and admit that if the above 12 points describe your lifestyle, then there is no need for you to take supplements. Now, you be honest and tell me who in this world today lives such a lifestyle?

## Supplement Categories

### Vitamins

Vitamins are organic substances necessary for life, which the body uses for essential body functions. Generally, the body cannot manufacture vitamins, so it must get them from food or supplements. While the body can live without a constant supply of all the vitamins, for optimal health all are necessary.

*Vitamins are not a replacement for food.*

Vitamins are not a replacement for food, and they do not give energy. Rather, they regulate our metabolism and provide the "spark" for our body to use enzymes and function on all "cylinders."

Most of the vitamins are designated by a letter of the alphabet and are generally divided into two categories: fat soluble, meaning they need fat for proper assimilation, and water soluble or water based.

### Fat Soluble Vitamins

*Vitamin A*

**Vitamin A:** Beneficial range: 10,000 to 50,000 IU.

Vitamin A can be supplied directly as vitamin A or in its pro vitamin form, known as carotene. The body can easily convert the pro vitamin into usable vitamin A.

Those who believe that high doses of vitamin A may be toxic, prefer carotene. Only very high amounts, over 50,000 units daily, show any real signs of possible toxicity.

Vitamin A is necessary for bones, teeth, skin and eyes (night blindness is considered a deficiency symptom). It helps resist infection and promotes healing. Vitamin A is recommended to treat acne, wrinkles, age spots, sore gums, emphysema and hyperthyroidism.

Natural Sources: Fish liver oil, carrots, green and yellow vegetables, dairy products and eggs.

*Vitamin D*

**Vitamin D:** Beneficial range: 400 to 1,200 IU.

Vitamin D may be acquired through sunlight on the skin or through diet. Necessary for healthy skin and bones, since it helps in the utilizing of calcium and phosphorus. Works well with calcium, vitamin C and vitamin A. Tooth decay, rickets and osteoporosis are considered to be deficiency symptoms. Night workers, people living in smog and northern climates should supplement vitamin D, especially in the winter. No doubt, this is why many of our mothers fed us cod-liver oil ( a rich source of vitamin A and D) in the winter time.

Natural Sources: Cod liver oil.

**Vitamin E:** Beneficial range 200 to 1,000 IU.

*Vitamin E*

Vitamin E is made up of eight compounds called toco-pherols, named after letters of the Greek alphabet. Alpha is the most important and is often the only one appearing in vitamin E supplements.

As an antioxidant, vitamin E prevents oxidation of fat compounds, protects the heart and the arteries, and acts as a vasodilator and anticoagulant. This vitamin is more effective working with selenium.

Vitamin E is considered to have anti-aging benefits. It helps to supply oxygen to the blood for more endurance, and protects the lungs from the damaging effects of pollution. It helps prevent blood clots and miscarriages, accelerates burn healing, and lowers the risk of heart disease.

Natural Sources: wheat germ, soybeans, vegetable oils, broccoli, leafy greens, whole grains and eggs.

**Vitamin F:** Beneficial Range: not established.

*Vitamin F*

Vitamin F is more commonly known as Unsaturated Fatty Acids, particularly linoleic and linolenic acid. It aids in preventing cholesterol deposits and promotes healthy skin and hair. It also may help to alleviate eczema, acne, and heart disease. (See also Chapter 9 under fats.)

Natural Sources: vegetable oils, sunflower seeds, soybeans, nuts and avocados.

**Vitamin K:** Beneficial Range: not established.

*Vitamin K*

The abundance of this vitamin in vegetables and oils makes vitamin K supplementation generally unnecessary. It is essential for blood clotting. Celiac disease, colitis, nosebleeds or excessive diarrhea may be deficiency symptoms.

### Water soluble vitamins

*Vitamin B Complex*

**The Vitamin B Complex:** The B vitamins are coenzymes which work most effectively as a team. They are involved in energy production and are helpful in alleviating depression and anxiety. They help maintain the health of the eyes, hair and skin as well as the liver, nerves and gastrointestinal tract. While they are best taken together, higher dosages of one may be taken if the need is there. Each of the B vitamins is discussed briefly below. Being water soluble, they must be daily replenished. Excess intake is easily excreted from the body.

*Vitamin B1
– thiamine*

**Vitamin B1 – thiamine:** Beneficial range: 10 - 100 mg.

B1 is needed to produce hydrochloric acid for digestion of carbohydrates. It promotes growth, improves mental attitude, affects energy and learning capacity, and keeps nerves, muscles and heart functioning normally.

Natural sources: brown rice, egg yolks, dried beans, whole grains, nuts and most vegetables.

*Vitamin B2
– riboflavin*

**Vitamin B2 – riboflavin:** Beneficial range: 10 - 100 mg.

B2 is necessary for red blood cell formation, for growth of skin, hair and nails. It alleviates eye fatigue and is important in prevention of cataracts. Deficiencies may be indicated by cracks and sores in the mouth and on the lips and skin. B2 is easily destroyed by light, cooking, antibiotics and alcohol.

Natural sources: Liver, kidney, cheese, milk, nuts and leafy, green vegetables.

*Vitamin B3
– niacin*

**Vitamin B3 – niacin, niacinamide:** Beneficial range: 50-500 mg.

B3 is needed for good circulation and healthy skin. It may reduce cholesterol, triglycerides, and high blood pressure, and can help to eliminate canker sores, migraine headaches and bad breath. Note: A harmless, warm, red flush may appear on the skin after taking niacin.

Natural sources: Beef, broccoli, potatoes, carrots, tomatoes, eggs, dates, figs, prunes and whole wheat.

**Vitamin B5 – pantothenic acid:** Beneficial range: 50 - 500 mg. B5 is important in the production of adrenal hormones and antibodies. This is why it is sometimes referred to as the anti-stress vitamin. It is used for the production of steroids and cortisone in the adrenal glands, and as well as in treating depression and anxiety.

*Vitamin B5 – pantothenic acid*

Natural Sources: beans, eggs, fish, fresh vegetables and whole wheat.

**Vitamin B6 – pyridoxine:** Beneficial range: 25 - 100 mg.

*Vitamin B6 – pyridoxine*

B6 is involved in many body functions. It must be present for the production of antibodies and red blood cells. It helps in the assimilation of protein and fats and reduces dry mouth, muscle spasms, leg cramps and hand numbness. B6 plays a role in cancer immunity, and in the treatment of allergies, arthritis, asthma and carpal tunnel syndrome.

Natural sources: Carrots, fish, eggs, peas, spinach, sunflower seeds, walnuts, wheat germ, soybeans, oats and cabbage.

**Vitamin B12 – cobalamin:** Beneficial range: 25 - 500 mcg.

*Vitamin B12 – cobalamin*

B12 is needed to prevent anemia because it is involved in forming and regenerating red blood cells. B12 is necessary for energy and fertility. It also helps to maintain concentration, memory, balance, and a healthy nervous system. It is poorly absorbed in the stomach, so a deficiency may appear when there is poor digestion or in the elderly.

Natural sources: Cheese, clams, eggs, milk, seafood, and tofu. B12 is found only in animal products, except for seaweed and spirulina. Vegetarians should take B12 supplements or be sure to eat spirulina or seaweed.

*Vitamin B15*
*– pangamic acid*

**Vitamin B15 – pangamic acid:** Beneficial range: not established.

B15 was made famous by the Russians who used it for athletic stamina and endurance. It is believed to extend the lifespan of cells, speed recovery from fatigue and aid in protein synthesis. It protects the liver, helps to overcome hangovers and may increase the blood's capacity to carry oxygen.

Natural sources: Brown rice, whole grains, sesame seeds and pumpkin seeds.

*Vitamin B17*
*– laetrile*

**Vitamin B17 – laetrile:** Beneficial range: Not over 1 gram.

This controversial "vitamin," derived from apricot pits, is believed by some to have cancer controlling benefits, but is considered illegal in Canada and the United States.

Natural sources: Seeds of apples, cherries, peaches, plums, apricots and nectarines.

*Folic acid*

**Folic acid:** Beneficial range: 200- 500 mcg.

Folic acid is essential to the formation of red blood cells and is sometimes considered a brain food. As a coenzyme in the synthesis of DNA, it is important for healthy cell division. Folic acid helps to prevent birth defects because it is essential for regulating embryonic and fetal development. Therefore, it is very important before and during pregnancy.

Natural sources: Deep green leafy vegetables, carrots, barley, beef, beans, bran, lamb, split peas, root vegetables and whole grains.

*PABA*

**PABA – para-aminobenzoic acid:** Beneficial range: 25-100 mg.

PABA helps form folic acid and assimilate protein. It protects against sunburn and skin cancer. PABA supplementation may restore gray hair to its natural color, if it was caused by stress or a deficiency.

Natural sources: Liver, kidney, whole grains, molasses, wheat germ and brown rice.

**Biotin:** Beneficial range: 25-200 mcg.                    *Biotin*

Biotin can be produced in the intestine, so deficiency is rare. It helps in cell growth, metabolism, and is necessary for healthy skin and hair. Vitamin C absorption requires biotin.

Natural sources: Milk, brown rice, soy and whole grains.

**Choline:** Beneficial range: 25 - 200 mg.                 *Choline*

Choline works with inositol to utilize fats and cholesterol. It regulates gallbladder and liver function. It is needed for nerve transmission and enhances brain function and memory. It may assist in disorders such as Parkinson's disease.

Natural sources: Meat, whole grains, green vegetables, nuts and lecithin.

**Inositol:** Beneficial range: 25-200 mg.                  *Inositol*

Inositol works with choline. It promotes hair growth, helps to prevent eczema, aids in the distribution of body fat, and nourishes brain cells.

Natural sources: Fruits, vegetables, peanuts and whole grains.

**Vitamin C – ascorbic acid:** Beneficial range: 500-3000 mg.      *Vitamin C*

Most animals have the ability to produce their own vitamin C, but humans, apes, and guinea pigs must rely on dietary sources. As an antioxidant, vitamin C plays a primary role in forming collagen which is necessary for the growth, repair and building of body tissues, cells, gums, blood vessels, bones and teeth. It helps lower cholesterol and absorb iron, but is used up more rapidly under stress or when smoking or elderly. Vitamin C passes out of the body within two or three hours, so high dosages should be spread throughout the day. To prevent or treat a common cold, take 500 mg. four to six times daily. Also, vitamin C can speed up wound healing. Easy bruising may be a deficiency symptom. Vitamin C is easily destroyed by light or heat.

Natural sources: Citrus fruits, fresh vegetables, berries, potatoes and peppers.

*Bioflavonoids*

**Bioflavonoids, also known as vitamin P**

Bioflavonoids work synergistically with vitamin C, and should be included in vitamin C supplements. They strengthen the walls of the capillaries.

Natural sources: White skin segment of citrus fruit, cherries, apricots and buckwheat.

## Minerals

### Major Minerals

These are needed in larger amounts than minor or trace minerals.

*Calcium*

**Calcium:** Beneficial range: 1000-2000 mg.

Calcium is the most abundant mineral in the human body. It is the major component of bones and teeth. It works with phosphorus for healthy bones and with magnesium for cardiovascular health. For calcium absorption, vitamin D must be available. Calcium is important for regular heartbeat, to alleviate insomnia, and to assist in nerve impulse transmission. Osteoporosis and cramping indicate a probable deficiency.

Natural sources: Dairy foods, sardines, seafood, green vegetables, almonds, kale, soybeans, asparagus, cabbage and sunflower seeds.

*Magnesium*

**Magnesium:** Beneficial range: 200-600 mg.

Magnesium is important for enzyme activity and assists in calcium, potassium, sodium and vitamin C uptake. It is necessary for the transmission of nerve and muscle impulses. It helps prevent depression, dizziness, muscle weakness, twitching and heart disease. It can relieve indigestion and work as a natural tranquilizer. Recent findings indicate that magnesium deficiency may be quite common.

Natural sources: Dairy foods, meat, whole grains, corn, nuts, dark green vegetables and bananas.

**Phosphorus:** Beneficial range: 1000-1500 mg.          *Phosphorus*

Phosphorus is needed for tooth and bone formation, cell growth, kidney function, nerve transmission, and the contraction of the heart muscle. It may help lessen the pain of arthritis. A proper balance of phosphorus, magnesium and calcium is important. Since phosphorus is abundant in foods, high dose supplementation is rarely needed.

Natural sources: Dairy foods, meat, fruit, legumes, vegetables and whole grains.

**Potassium:** Beneficial range: 100-500 mg. elemental.          *Potassium*

Potassium works as a regulator for heartbeat, blood pressure, the nervous system, kidneys and water balance. Sodium and potassium balance is important. Too much sodium may frustrate potassium absorption.

Natural sources: Fruit, tomatoes, green vegetables, sunflower seeds, bananas, potatoes, and nuts.

**Sodium:** Beneficial range: 1000-3000 mg.          *Sodium*

Supplementation is considered to be rarely necessary. Sodium is important for maintaining proper water balance and blood pH. It is also involved in stomach, muscle and nerve function, and helps to keep calcium and other minerals in the blood soluble. Sodium and potassium must be kept in proper balance, and since sodium is much more prevalent in the average diet, potassium supplementation is more advisable.

Natural sources: Most foods contain sodium, kelp is especially high.

### Minor minerals

Chromium

**Chromium:** Beneficial range: 50-250 mcg.

Chromium is involved with insulin in the metabolism of sugar, so it is needed for energy. It also helps lower high blood pressure, and works as a deterrent for diabetes.

Natural sources: Brown rice, wheat germ, corn, dried beans, mushrooms and potatoes.

Copper

**Copper:** Beneficial range: 1-4 mg.

Copper is required to convert the body's iron into hemoglobin. It aids in the formation of bones, red blood cells and works with vitamin C and zinc to form elastin. Osteoporosis may be an early deficiency sign.

Natural sources: Almonds, avocados, barley, peas, wheat, nuts and soybeans.

Iodine

**Iodine:** Beneficial range: 100- 300 mcg.

Iodine is integral in thyroid function and controls metabolism. A lack of this mineral can result in slow mental function, weight gain and a lack of energy. Some believe that iodine deficiency may be linked to breast cancer.

Natural sources: Seafood, kelp, onions, asparagus, lima beans, mushrooms and soybeans.

Iron

**Iron:** Beneficial range: 10-50 mg.

Iron is often poorly absorbed in the body. Pregnant and menstruating women need higher amounts. Iron is needed for the production of hemoglobin and the oxygenation of red blood cells. It is the blood's most abundant mineral. It aids in growth and helps to prevent disease and fatigue. A primary deficiency symptom is iron deficiency anemia. Amounts over 2 grams can be fatal to small children. Since iron can accumulate in the body, becoming toxic, high dosages should be taken only under supervision.

Natural sources: Organ meats, egg yolks, nuts, beans, millet, parsley, peaches, pears and pumpkins.

**Manganese:** Beneficial range: 5-50 mg. *Manganese*

Manganese plays a part in protein, blood carbohydrate and fat production, and sugar regulation. It is necessary for healthy nerves and brain, sex hormone production, normal skeletal development and a healthy immune system. It helps to reduce fatigue, prevent osteoporosis, and reduce nervous irritability.

Natural sources: Whole grains, nuts, peas, beans, leafy green vegetables, blueberries and pineapples.

**Selenium:** Beneficial range: 10-100 mcg. *Selenium*

Selenium is an important antioxidant that works synergistically with vitamin E by strengthening the immune system and preventing the formation of damaging free radicals. This gives it a frontline cancer prevention function. Along with vitamin E, it also helps to maintain a healthy heart.

A deficiency of selenium may result in muscle breakdown and a weak heart. This is why newborn lambs and calves are often given an immediate dose of selenium. Since many soils are depleted in selenium, supplementation is advisable.

Natural sources: Brazil nuts, broccoli, brown rice, tomatoes, whole grains, and onions (depending on amount in the soil).

**Sulphur:** Beneficial range: Supplementation rarely necessary. *Sulphur*

Sulphur is essential for healthy hair, skin and nails. It disinfects the blood, resists bacteria, stimulates bile secretions and protects against toxic substances. As it keeps the hair shiny, the skin soft and supple and is thought to slow down the aging process, it is sometimes referred to as the "beauty mineral".

Natural sources: Cabbage, beans, brussels sprouts, garlic, onions and turnips.

*Zinc*

**Zinc:** Beneficial range: 15-50 mg.

Zinc is important for disease fighting, wound healing and protecting the immune system. It is important in prostrate and brain function, helps in formation of insulin, and plays a role in taste and smelling ability. White marks on fingernails are regarded as zinc deficiency symptoms.

Natural sources: Seafood, oysters, whole grains, pumpkin seeds, sunflower seeds, soybeans, pecans, and mushrooms.

### Trace minerals

There are up to 70 trace minerals, 40 of which may be necessary for optimal health. The amounts necessary are very small and generally not precisely known. Some may be necessary in minute amounts but harmful in large amounts. Some may be dangerous or even fatal. A few of the most well-known are as follows.

*Aluminium*

**Aluminium:** There is no established function for aluminium in the body, but it can have destructive effects. It weakens the living tissue of the alimentary canal (digestive tract), and destroys vitamins. It can cause colic, nausea, skin ailments, loss of memory, and may be a significant contributor to Alzheimer's disease and Lou Gehrig's disease. It can be found in tap water, table salt (added to prevent caking), foil, cookware, antiperspirants, baking powder, processed cheeses and bleached flour.

All efforts should be made to limit exposure to aluminium.

*Boron*

**Boron:** Boron is needed in small amounts for calcium absorption in the body. Elderly people may benefit from 2 to 3 mg. daily supplementation. It is found in leafy green vegetables, nuts and grains.

**Fluorine:** Fluoride, the active form of fluorine, is the focus of much controversy. Proponents claim that it reduces tooth decay and strengthens bones, and have successfully influenced many cities to add it to drinking water. Opponents point out that it is both a deadly poison and destructive to the immune system and that we already get more than adequate amounts from foods. From my experience I strongly recommend avoiding fluoride, in any form, including in toothpaste.

*Fluorine*

**Germanium:** Some researcher have claimed that germanium plays an important role in immune function. They believe it helps the body recover from many illnesses such as rheumatoid arthritis, cholesterol, viral infections and cancer. It is very expensive because only minute amounts are found in plants. Trace amounts are found in aloe vera, ginseng, shitake mushrooms and onions.

*Germanium*

**Molybdenum:** This essential trace element is needed in very small quantities. It enables the body to use nitrogen and is also necessary for urine production. It is found in whole grains and dark, leafy green vegetables.

*Molybdenum*

**Nickel:** Nickel is an essential trace mineral and may be a factor in RNA and DNA stabilization. Nickel is a by-product of industry and is found in heating fuel, automobile exhaust and cigarette smoke. Toxicity from excess is more probable than deficiency. It is also found in seafood, grains, beans and vegetables. Ear piercing, especially in children, may contribute to nickel toxicity.

*Nickel*

*Silicon*

**Silicon:** Silicon is present in bone and connective tissue and is important for collagen formation. It is needed for healthy skin, nails and hair, and plays a significant role in preventing cardiovascular disease. Foods that contain silicon include alfalfa, beets, horsetail herb, soybeans, green vegetables and whole grains.

*Vanadium*

**Vanadium:** Vanadium is present in most body tissues and is needed for cell metabolism and for the forming of bones and teeth. It plays a role in growth and reproduction. A vanadium deficiency may be linked to cardiovascular and kidney disease, and impaired reproductive ability. Vanadium is easily destroyed in food processing. It is found in fish, vegetable oils, radishes, whole grains and olives.

### Colloidal Minerals

In recent years extensive publicity has drawn attention to what are referred to as colloidal minerals. (Colloidal minerals are not another category but rather a form of minerals.) These are relatively large electrically neutral mineral crystals that remain suspended in water. To what degree these elements can be utilized by the body has not yet been fully determined. Evidence suggests that glacier and naturally mineralized water, such as concentrated sea source minerals, do carry an electrical charge and are more easily assimilated by the body.

### Microclusters

Microclusters contain an entirely new type of mineral colloids referred to as "nanocolloids™." These crystals, discovered and patented by Drs. Patrick and Gael Crystal Flanagan as Flanagan Microclusters® (available under the name of Crystal Energy®), are only 1/1000 the size of typical mineral colloids and contain a powerful electrical charge referred to as zeta potential.

Because of their smallness and electrical charge, they enhance the wetting ability of water by breaking down its surface tension. This allows the water, and whatever it carries, to be more easily absorbed by the body. Since all food is carried into body tissues by water, adding Crystal Energy® has been shown to increase body hydration and enhance absorption of nutrients.

## Fats

In spite of the bad press that fat has been getting in recent years, fat is required and used by the human body in numerous ways. Fat is used in manufacturing antibodies to fight disease. It acts as carriers for the fat soluble vitamins A, D, E and K. Fat deposits also cushion, protect and hold in place vital organs such as the liver, kidneys and the heart. Fat is the body's insulation against temperature changes and gives our body its shape. It is one of three energy sources; it aids in digestion and produces a satisfying feeling of fullness after a meal. From these reasons alone, it should be obvious that it is not wise to try to eliminate all fats from our diet. There are two types of fat in the body:

*For more on fats see also page 114.*

1. Nonessential fats are those which our body is able to manufacture.

2. Essential fats are the fats which the body cannot make and must be made available through our diet. These are necessary for healthy skin, growth, blood; arteries and nerves. They also help to keep our metabolism running smoothly. Adults need at least 15 to 25 grams of dietary fat daily to meet the body's need.

### Polyunsaturated Fats

Polyunsaturated fats are found in most foods, but mainly in fish, nuts, oils from plants, seeds and soybeans. These oils are liquid at room temperature and help to reduce blood cholesterol.

### Mono-unsaturated Fats

Mono-unsaturated fats are found in most foods, but mainly in vegetable and nut oils such as olive, peanut and canola oil. These also remain liquid at room temperature and reduce blood cholesterol.

### Hydrogenated Fats

Both of the above unsaturated fats can be hydrogenated, by adding hydrogen, in order to make them solid at room temperature and thus more usable in the processing of foods such as baked goods, nondairy creamers and whipped toppings. Some nutritionists consider this an adulteration and suggest, as I would that they be best avoided.

### Saturated Fats

This includes all animal source fats such as meats, dairy, including cheese, milk and ice cream. Coconut, palm, cocoa butter (as in chocolate) are also saturated fats. These fats raise blood cholesterol and should be consumed as little as possible.

A much higher percentage of calories from fat are stored as body fat than the calories from carbohydrates and protein. Because of this, calories from protein and carbohydrates are much less prone to contribute to obesity.

## Carbohydrates

Carbohydrates are the body's main source of the energy necessary for body heat and function. They are essential for brain and nervous system function and also assist in the digestion and assimilation of food. During digestion, starches and sugars, the principal kinds of carbohydrates, are broken down into glucose (also known as blood sugar), which then provides energy.

If one does not get enough carbohydrate, protein, which should be available for building body tissue, will need to be used for energy. If we eat too many carbohydrates, more than needed for glucose and glycogen, the body will store it up as fat. When the body needs more fuel, the fat can be converted back to glucose and some weight may be lost. Rather than getting lost in technical details, let's simplify the matter of carbohydrates by putting it into the following categories.

*Glycogen: extra glucose stored in the liver and muscles.*

### Complex Carbohydrates

Complex carbohydrates are found in grains, beans, corn, peas, leafy green vegetables, tubers, potatoes, onions and turnips. These carbohydrates, being complex, take much longer for the body to digest and turn into usable fuel. Therefore, they burn longer and more steadily, putting much less stress on the body's blood sugar control mechanism. Consumed in moderation, they have little tendency to cause obesity.

### Simple Carbohydrates

Simple carbohydrates are the sugars found in fruits, fruit juices, white flour and white rice. Although these give quick energy, they digest quickly and cause stress to the glandular and hormonal systems of the body. They should be eaten separately and in relatively small amounts. Heavy consumption of simple carbohydrates can raise triglycerides, aggravate blood sugar problems and cause weight gain.

### Refined Carbohydrates

Refined carbohydrates are, in effect, simple carbohydrates that have been processed, stripped of nutrients and fiber and intensified in sweetness. (They are sometimes referred to as empty calories.) All forms of sugar, honey, maple sugar, concentrated fruit juices, barley malt and even white flour fall into this category. The human body was made to handle such "intense" carbohydrates only in emergency. When they become a routine part of the diet, the stress on the body will greatly increase the tendency for diabetes, obesity, immune breakdown and the susceptibility for disease.

## Protein

*For more on protein in our diet see Chapter 9.*

Next to water, protein is the most abundant element in the body. Protein is made up of amino acids which are sometimes referred to as the building blocks that provide the structure for all living things. In the human body, protein makes up the muscles, ligaments, tendons, organs, glands, hair, nails and body fluids. Protein is needed to convey certain minerals throughout the body and has countless other functions. It becomes easy to see why it was given the name "pro-tein" which means "of first importance."

### Amino Acids

The total protein complex contains approximately 22 to 29 (depending on which expert you ask) amino acids. All of these must be available at the same time for the body to derive the full benefit of protein. About 80 percent of these amino acids can be manufactured by the human liver; the remaining ones, called essential amino acids, must be supplied by the food consumed.

### Essential Amino Acids

*See Chapter 9.*

The essential amino acids (about eight in number) are those which the body cannot make, but must receive from an outside food source. Foods such as eggs, meat, dairy, soybeans and spirulina, which contain all of the essential amino acids, are referred to as complete proteins. Only small amounts of the above are needed at any one time, and a complete protein is also possible without animal foods.

## Enzymes

The thousands of known enzymes play a role in virtually all bodily activities. Each enzyme has a specific function in the body that no other enzyme can fill. No mineral, vitamin or hormone could do any work without the presence of enzymes. Some enzymes are found in plants; others are made by the pancreas. They cannot be manufactured synthetically. Of the numerous enzyme active in the body, we will look primarily at the digestive enzymes, since, if these are adequate, others will probably be okay.

*Enzymes are easily destroyed by heat and processing.*

### Digestive Enzymes

There are about twenty-two digestive enzymes, which are necessary to digest protein, carbohydrates, sugars and fats. Enzymes begin digesting food in the mouth. In the stomach, additional enzymes begin working and continue the digestive process. As the food enters the upper intestine, the pancreas provides pancreatic enzymes to further break down the food. Still more enzymes work to deliver nutrients to the cells of the body.

Enzymes, which naturally occur in plants, are easily destroyed by heat and processing. When this happens, the body's capacity to produce enzymes is overtaxed, and digestion is frustrated. This causes gas and inefficient use of food nutrients. Fresh, whole and especially green foods, as well as green phytonutrient powders are important to assure adequate enzyme levels.

The main digestive enzymes are amylase, protase, lipase, pepsin and hydrochloric acid. Amylase, found in saliva, breaks down carbohydrates. This is why it is so important to chew our food well. Protase, found in the stomach juices, helps to digest protein. Lipase aids in the digestion of fats, as does bile, which is a secretion of the liver. Pepsin is another protein digesting enzyme secreted out of the stomach wall.

Hydrochloric acid in the stomach digests protein, calcium and iron. When eating under stress, the secretion of hydrochloric acid is reduced and indigestion is common.

Enzyme supplementation and enzyme therapy show great potential in enhancing digestion and general health improvement. I believe they will become an increasingly more important part of help yourself health care.

### Coenzymes

The study of coenzymes is relatively new. Coenzyme Q10 (CoQ10) has been studied the most. It shows great promise as a supplement and is known to have anti-aging benefits. It is especially helpful for improving heart function. CoQ10 has also been found to stimulate the production of insulin.

## Phytonutrients

*Supplements especially important for those not getting fresh, live green foods.*

Phytonutrients or phytochemicals are a relatively new concept sometimes referred to as being part of the "green revolution." Green foods contain chlorophyll, as well as many vital enzymes and chemicals yet to be discovered and named. These ingredients are very important for optimal health. This is why many people who have been taking green supplements, such as barley green, wheat grass, green kamut or spirulina have seen dramatic health improvements.

I am convinced that this form of supplementation will become very popular. It is especially important for those who are not consistently eating fresh, live green foods.

## Herbs

In a most general sense, herbs are any plants that are conducive to maintaining or regaining health. According to the book of Genesis, all plants were given to man for food or medicine. For our purposes, we will comment briefly on herbs in the following three categories.

### General or Primary

These herbs are plants which are acceptable for regular and continuous consumption. Many of them are known to be rich in certain minerals or vitamins: carrots are rich in beta carotene; beets are rich in iron; cabbage is rich in vitamin K. Since antioxidants, especially vitamin C, are very necessary for good health, many of the general or complementary herbs contain them in abundance, and healthy are those who eat them regularly.

*Herbs are amongst nature's greatest treasures.*

### Remedial

Here, I would include those plants which are relatively harmless, but not needed or advised for consumption on a regular basis as a primary food. They may be unique in having a specific effect on the human physiology and may cause the body to react in a definite way: dandelion root may have a purging effect on the liver; walnut hulls may have an anti-parasite effect; chamomile may be a mild sedative. While these herbs are not potentially harmful, they should be used with moderation and with some degree of knowledge.

Some herbs such as garlic, aloe vera, ginger, etc. can be healthful even if used daily, although they would probably never become a primary source of food like those above.

This category of herbs is a rich part of the legacy of our ancestors. It is sad that we have not had this awareness handed down to us as a part of personal health maintenance inheritance. It is even more shameful that governments and medical monopolists are working aggressively to rob us of this heritage and are already moving to make the sale and use of these herbs illegal. We must do everything possible to resist this effort to usurp our capacity to take responsibility for our own health.

This category certainly does not include herbs like comfrey or hawthorne, which have been safely used by millions for thousands of years.

### Medicinal

No doubt, there are herbs which may be helpful, but which also have been clearly demonstrated to be potentially harmful. These may be restricted, or at least only allowed to be sold and/ or promoted by persons qualified to handle them. This category might include herbs like lobelia.

Hopefully the above will serve as a basic primer for all who wish to get a basic understanding of elements for good health and general supplementation.

# Chapter 12

# *Elimination*

Proper elimination is as important as that of supply for a healthy life. Many nutrition writers and advisors take it for granted, and most others treat it only in a casual way. Then, there are those who make it everything. We will attempt to show how it belongs along side of good nutrition as a practical daily way to maintain or regain good health.

I mentioned earlier about my response to the question regarding when I got into nutrition (Moments after birth and ever since, of course!). I might have continued the story. Soon after she gave me a supply of nutrition, my mother had another challenge. A significant amount of the supply had resurfaced. Being a wise and experienced mom, she accepted this as an encouraging sign, and only when elimination was not proper did she become concerned.

## Two Aspects of Elimination

### Discarding Residual Debris

Only a part of the food we eat contains nutritional value for our bodies. Much of food acts as a vehicle or container for the vital elements (i.e. vitamins, minerals, enzymes, fats, protein, phytochemicals, etc.). Fiber is the primary vehicle. It is necessary for peristaltic action and bowel function. Digestion is the process of converting the vital elements into a usable form. Absorption and assimilation is the process of extracting these elements, transferring them into the blood stream and sending them to the various organs. The unusable elements or the elements that act as carriers must be eliminated. This waste, also known as feces, must be eliminated promptly and regularly.

Metabolism and other body processes also produce waste materials. Cells die and must be discarded and replaced. If allowed to accumulate, excess bile and other metabolic waste becomes toxic and destructive to our health. We all are detoxifying our bodies daily. If we detoxify too slowly, we become chronically ill and will eventually die because of the accumulation of internal sewage.

### Environmental Contaminants

The above aspect is more or less what our ancestors' bodies had to deal with. However, a whole new soup of contaminants is assaulting our bodies every day. This soup includes chemicals and environmental pollutants which enter our bodies through food, water and air. This toxic mixture must be discharged promptly and entirely. Without a doubt, the abundance of such elements, and the slow or partial elimination of the same, lies behind much of our health breakdown today. In fact, here may lie the elusive cause of the cancer that is destroying human lives in ever-increasing numbers.

*This toxic mixture must be discharged promptly and entirely.*

## Pollution is Everywhere

We all have become aware that our environment has become polluted. We didn't used to see the air we breathed or smell the water we drank! The food we ate didn't used to include ingredients that we couldn't even pronounce.

The danger of additives, preservatives and agricultural chemicals is assessed by how much the human body can tolerate on a given day. However, the effects of the accumulation of these toxic substances in the body are neither known nor considered. Now we are beginning to realize that a poorly nourished and under exercised body does tend to accumulate toxicity. As a result, we not only exist with a polluted environment around us, but also carry a polluted "invironment" within us!

*Lack of fiber and a diet of processed food causes the colon to become congested and inefficient in its food use. This can result in malnutrition, colitis and other chronic diseases.*

This toxic load becomes a generator of free radicals. Free radicals are unattached chemical entities which latch onto cells and frustrate normal cellular duplication. This sets the stage for ill health, even cancer, and immune breakdown.

Polluting elements may also aggravate joints and muscle function and lead to arthritic, muscular problems and heart disease.

So, in today's highly polluted environment, supporting the body's cleansing and detoxifying functions has become almost indispensable for maintaining good health. In fact, many have recovered from chronic health challenges after taking these suggested steps for body cleansing and detoxification.

## Normal Detoxification

Besides adequate nutritional intake, the human body requires elimination. Stale, used air is exhaled through breathing. The sweat glands and the kidneys work to eliminate polluted water. The bowels work to process and pass bacteria and unusable food stuff. These are the body's routine, normal cleansing and detoxifying processes. If any of the organs involved do not function, the body quickly becomes toxic and disease soon runs rampant.

Our body is designed to be self-detoxifying. An understanding of our eliminating organs is important for us to be able to facilitate rather than frustrate detoxification.

*Our body is designed to be self-detoxifying.*

### The Lungs

Our lungs function not only to absorb oxygen but also to detoxify the body. When the blood enters the lungs, it releases toxic gases which then are eliminated by the lungs as we exhale. Keeping our lungs clean and efficient is crucial to good health. One of the great benefits of exercise is that the lungs are stimulated. To keep your lungs in good shape, practice deep breathing and avoid breathing all frustrations such as fumes, chemicals, smoke or inhalants.

*Keeping our lungs clean and efficient is crucial to good health.*

### The Skin

Few are aware that the skin is a major eliminating organ of the human body. A great amount of toxic waste is eliminated through the skin, especially through the sweat glands. This is a strong reason to encourage sweating rather than trying to avoid or frustrate this natural process. This is also why I strongly discourage the use of antiperspirants. Not only do they restrict an important eliminating function, but also they contain aluminium which is very toxic and does not belong on the human body.

I believe that the use of antiperspirants may be a direct contributing factor to the dramatic rise in the incidence of breast cancer and may also be implicated in Alzheimer's. Find and use a good natural deodorant. Remember, a body that is clean on the inside does not have a bad odor. An antiperspirant makes as much sense as an invention to restrict urination or bowel movements!

Skin diseases, boils, rashes and itching may all be evidence of a toxic body which is being frustrated in its normal elimination process. Instead of trying to find a cream to suppress this expression, activate elimination and allow a natural recovery.

### The Kidneys

*Drink more water.*

The importance of kidney function in elimination is generally overlooked, at least until the kidneys are destroyed. At that time the person may suddenly find himself on dialysis to remove the deadly toxins which are no longer being removed naturally. All of the blood passes through these filtering organs which remove uric acid, toxins and myriads of harmful chemicals. To do this job effectively requires a lot of liquid. This is a strong reason for drinking more water.

A relative of ours had a serious head injury and was permanently put on strong medications for serious headaches. After a number of years it was discovered that his kidneys were being destroyed by the medication. His body became seriously toxic and required dialysis, a process where the blood is artificially filtered to take out the toxic waste which the kidneys would normally remove.

Eventually, a kind sister donated a kidney. Before the operation, they kept him on dialysis for a good cleansing. They installed the kidney, and by the time the patient was conscious, the real kidney was filtering the blood ten times better than the artificial dialysis kidney. Now, his health is better, but he must always take drugs to suppress his immune system so that it does not reject the donated kidney. This suppressing of his immune system makes him very susceptible to infection and disease. Our kidneys are definitely worth protecting.

Drinking plenty of water and taking the natural way for health care is the best kidney protection plan.

*Disease often evolves as a result of neglecting and abusing the colon.*

### The Bowels (Colon)

The most obvious eliminating organ is our bowel. While it is obvious, too often it is taken for granted, until as happens to thousands, colon and rectal disease (including cancer) strikes. Actually disease does not strike. It evolves as a result of neglecting and abusing this most lowly servant of our body's function. Highly respected health pioneers such as Dr. Norman Walker, Dr. Bernard Jensen, Dr. William Kellogg, and Victor Irons all have concluded that bowel neglect probably lies at the root of most health breakdown.

What house can be clean if the waste system is not functioning? What city can be healthy if the garbage is not being removed? Our own waste system is just as crucial to our health.

Here again is a strong reason for drinking more water, but also a reason for eating fiber rich foods and avoiding sticky, gooey "paste-ry" and dead white bread. A healthy body must have at least one, preferably more, easy bowel movements daily. If this is not your case, adjust your diet or supplement it with herbs such as cascara sagrada, flax seed, psyllium husk, wheat bran or prunes.

*Irrigation – see Dr. Jensen's book in Bibliography.*

No doubt, with the extra work our bowel is required to do for us in our present lifestyle, bowel management, including colon cleansing and irrigation, may serve a health enhancing purpose. This lowly servant will serve you well if you care for it and provide it with the water, food and fiber it needs!

### Reduce Pollution Intake

Not only must we stop the pollution of the environment around us, but even more immediate is the need to stop polluting our bodies. Processing food not only devitalizes and robs the food of many essential elements, but also adds chemical preservatives, flavorings and colorings which in turn add to the body's toxic load. Avoiding processed foods as well as coffee, pop and other drinks containing caffeine can be a healthy step away from internal pollution.

We must become as concerned about internal pollution as we are about environmental pollution. You may be able to move to a cleaner environment, but how can you move to a cleaner body?

## Practice Detoxification

While we take steps to reduce our intake of polluting elements, we can also begin to rid ourselves of accumulated toxicity and health robbing internal debris. Eating fresh raw foods, whole grains and adequate fiber, and drinking clean pure water are all important for ridding the body of internal pollution.

· *fresh raw foods*
· *whole grains*
· *adequate fiber*
· *clean pure water*

For centuries man has found herbs, clay, certain juices, as well as fasting to be helpful for stimulating the body's natural cleansing processes. Recent studies and experimentation have found that the proper use of these things can still be effective to rid the body of even today's internal pollution. Such cleansing has helped many whose health was failing to regain normal good health.

## A Specific Cleansing Program

Imagine a fourteen day experience during which toxicity is drawn from the body and brought into the colon. Then this toxic accumulation and the longtime mucous encrustation and waste in the colon is removed as a painless but colorful display of debris. All this can be accomplished at home during normal routine with minimum discomfort. The result will be a new vim and vigor, and a "clean" inner bill of health.

I have developed a two week cleansing program which has been used by tens of thousands of people. Many of them declare that it was the pivotal factor that finally arrested their health deterioration. It is fully described in my book, *Healthy Steps.* The actual program is available in packaged form from Royal BodyCare (in the USA 1-800-722-0444 or in Canada 1-800-567-5433).

The fourteen days are divided into three periods. The first seven days are the preparation phase. During this time, one takes two daily portions of herbs and supplements which activate a general body detoxification. Toxins, heavy metals, and other pollutants are drawn from the cells and dumped into the colon.

*Regular, spring, and fall cleaning for a clean house ...*

The second phase, lasting four days, is the actual colon cleanse. During this time, besides taking two portions of supplements, four doses of clay-psyllium powder mixed with juices are ingested. This, plus other liquids, are taken in place of solid food. Avoiding solid food allows the mix to soften and loosen debris and encrustation from the intestinal and colon walls. The clay attracts and holds the toxins in suspension and the psyllium bulk moves the entire mess out of the body. If the term "good riddance" is ever appropriate, it certainly is in this case.

The third phase, referred to as the restoration time, supplies two daily portions of supplements. These, including acidophilus and digestive enzymes, resupply the internal organs to develop an ideal atmosphere for good digestion and absorption.

My mother told us as children, "Besides regular cleaning, spring and fall house cleaning are the secret for a clean house." I believe this is also good advice for keeping a clean and healthy body.

# Chapter 13

# *The Immune System*

One of the most fascinating and amazing aspects of the human body is the immune system. Without it we would be as defenseless as a rabbit hopping around in a rifle range. The genius behind this wonderful surveillance and defence system is far beyond human wisdom. Since it is our around-the-clock indispensable protector, we certainly should know a little about it, especially how we can encourage and help it in its life-preserving work. Should it shut down, we would be as defenseless as a person in the last stages of AIDS.

*The genius behind this wonderful surveillance and defence system is far beyond human wisdom.*

## Numerous Lines of Defence

We have many weapons to protect us. Our skin and mucous membranes create a barrier to insulate us from invasion. Our skin also has secretions that kill many germs while we are alive – this capacity is lost at death, and this is why cadavers take on ugly colors. Our digestive juices are so highly acidic that they can dissolve germs. Fevers burn up microorganisms; special cells such as macrophages, T-cells, killer cells, B-cells and antibodies attack and devour intruders.

We also have an internal defense industry that produces armaments. The bone marrow, spleen, thymus, tonsils, adenoids, appendix, and lymph nodes all play a part in equipping this amazingly competent and complete weapons system.

## The Workings of the Immune System

*Our immune system patrols every part of our body.*

We will explain the immune system only briefly and in a very basic, simple way. Consider that it patrols every cell of our body. It surveys every element that contacts or enters our body to determine if it is acceptable. If it is living tissue, it must be our own or it will be immediately rejected. This is why skin grafts must be from our own body, and why organ transplants have a major problem with rejection. If a virus, bacteria, splinter, dead cell or even a cancer cell is detected, it must be appropriately marked and destroyed or at least isolated so that it cannot harm our healthy cells.

*Our bodies might be exposed to as many virus and bacteria in a month as our ancestors faced in an average lifetime.*

With modern travel and constant social contact, our bodies might be exposed to as many virus and bacteria in a month as our ancestors faced in an average lifetime. With the added frustration of so many chemicals in our environment (preservatives, colorings, flavorings and additives in our food and pollutants in our air and water), our immune systems must certainly work overtime.

## The Battle with Invaders

When a bacteria gets a slight advantage and an infection results, the immune system needs some time to catch up. A rise in body temperature often is required to help to destroy the infected cells. Meanwhile, the host, with inadequate knowledge and absolutely no patience, rushes off to get an antibiotic. While the antibiotic may reduce recovery time, it compromises the immune system, destroys positive bacteria in the gut, and provides yet another opportunity for the invading bacteria to develop resistance.

If instead of antibiotics, some antioxidants were taken and the immune system's activity was reinforced, the recovery would be natural. With this approach, however, our immune system would gain more experience, broaden its immune capacity and be instantly ready should such bacteria attempt another attack.

*While the antibiotic may reduce recovery time, it compromises the immune system.*

During my childhood, my father refused vaccinations until they became legally required. Whenever one of us eight children contracted a childhood disease, my mother would have the rest of us sleep with the sick one. Within a few weeks, the entire lot of us had measles, mumps, chicken pox or whatever was going on. After this we were immune, my mother had peace, and life could go on. Mom didn't understand the science of how the immune system stored all this information in its memory so that it could instantly react the next time it encountered that disease. She knew, however, that once we had had it, that sickness would rarely ever have a chance to get through the immune defences a second time.

*For more on vaccinations, see Chapter 15.*

In contrast, today, even though most children have been vaccinated, if the disease strikes some years later, they may again be at risk and so require another vaccination. For more on vaccinations pro and con, see the bibliography.

## Cancer and Autoimmune Disease

Every cell in our body must be replaced in an identical form in order for life to continue. When you bite your tongue and destroy some tongue cells, you do not want them to be replaced by liver or toenail cells.

Our body replaces dead cells through a process called cell division. This process goes on continually and is governed by blueprints called RNA and DNA within the nucleus of each cell. When toxins or free radicals invade the cells, they may alter the RNA/DNA codes. The result is an abnormal or mutant cell. Each time this mutant cell divides, it will produce another mutant cell which will produce another mutant cell and – well, you get the point. Sometimes, one or more of these cells begins to divide erratically. Instead of reproducing one new cell, it produces hundreds of cells – all abnormal like itself. These abnormal cells, clustered together, form a tumor. The first stages in the development of cancer are now in process.

*If our immune system is working effectively, the mutant cells will be detected and destroyed.*

Terrifying? Yes, it is, but the process just described is happening dozens of times each hour, in your body and in mine.

If our immune system is working effectively, it will detect this abnormal situation. The mutant cells will be isolated and destroyed, and thus the immune system will deal with the problem, and a healthy life can continue.

Since the immune system is capable of guarding against and conquering cancerous cells, the most logical way to deal with cancer is to intensify this protective activity. When cancer is overcome in this way, it is truly a miracle of remission. Once we appreciate how the immune system works, it should be clear that the best way to prevent cancer is to keep our bodies well nourished, internally clean, and defensively strong. This brings us back to the A SED theory as explained earlier.

*... to prevent cancer keep body well nourished, internally clean, and defensively strong.*

Autoimmune disease is a condition where the immune system seems to become disoriented and begins to attack "friendly" tissue or otherwise harmless elements. If this autoimmune attack occurs in the upper respiratory tract, wheezing, sniffing and sneezing, as in hay fever, often develop. When it occurs in the skin region, welts, hives, itching and swelling may result. This is the basic dynamic behind common allergies.

The most severe form of autoimmune disease occurs when the immune system begins to attack its own host. Rheumatoid arthritis for example is where the body's immune cells begin to attack the joints. Lupus and multiple sclerosis are other examples of autoimmune related diseases.

## Care and Support for the Immune System

The immune system is available to protect or carry us through abnormal situations. In order to do this effectively, it must be maintained in good condition and be well supplied, especially when it is on active duty. Like an army, it is available on standby to rally at times of crisis, but it was never designed to be furiously engaged in all-out battle continuously.

Presently, due to a constant onslaught of chemicals, pollutants, electromagnetic frequencies, and endless other "stressors," most immune systems are engaged in all-out battle continuously. Besides this total combat engagement, the immune system is often poorly supplied, undernourished and working in unsanitary conditions. No wonder it gets confused, as in autoimmune response, or unable to overcome carcinogenic elements as in the case of cancer!

*The immune system was never designed to be furiously engaged in all-out battle continuously*

Here again I can only reiterate once more: keep your body well nourished; keep it clean and keep your defense system strong. To activate and empower the immune system, there are certain foods, herbs, supplements and superfoods, which can be helpful. I list some examples below.

### Foods

Greens such as broccoli, kale, cabbage, spinach and cauliflower. Carotenoids as found in green and orange fruits and vegetables. Mushrooms, soybeans, garlic, apples, oranges, apricots and berries.

### Herbs

Licorice root, echinacea, pau d'arco, goldenseal, and kelp.

### Supplements

Antioxidants: vitamins A, C and E, selenium, pantothenic acid, zinc, acidophilus, CoQ10, germanium and all minerals.

### Superfoods

Spirulina, aloe vera, Crystal Energy®, barley green, all phyto-nutrients containing chlorophyll.

# Chapter 14

# Nutrition for Pregnancy and Pre-Conception

## *by Ron Zehr*

The health of a child should be a concern to parents long before the first incident of fever, flu or runny nose. More and more, we are learning that many of the health problems encountered later in childhood and even into adulthood are simply the harvest of innocuous seeds planted in those first formative years.

I am appalled when I see the food offered to children. I am shocked when I witness the diets of nursing and pregnant women. I am saddened when I see the eating habits of "wannabe" and "gonnabe" parents.

*Our starting point must always be the health of the parents.*

While it is important to consider health for children, our starting point must always be the health of the parents – yes, I did say parents, as in both mother and father. They are both responsible for the health of their children.

## Preconception

The responsibility of bringing a new life into existence is an awesome one. Some have said that a couple should begin preparing for pregnancy at least two years before conception. The health of the embryo, the fetus, the baby, the child and even the adult that will come from that conception may be significantly affected by the health of both parents.

*The rising incidence of infertility should come as a warning to us.*

The rising incidence of infertility, particularly in the western world, should come as a warning to us. The rising incidence of babies developing or even being born with serious health problems should make all of us sit up and take notice.

While it is obvious that both a woman's egg and a man's sperm are necessary for conception, it should be equally obvious that both contribute to the health of the child which will develop from that conception. If either the egg or the sperm is seriously unhealthy, fertilization and conception cannot occur. Even if the egg and sperm are healthy enough for fertilization to occur, they may not be able to produce a healthy embryo, and the mother may miscarry or the child born may have health problems that manifest themselves from birth or which crop up later in life.

Generally, the health of the sperm or egg is a reflection of the health of the man or woman. It is vital then, that both would-be parents are acquainted with the perspectives, and apply the practices in this book. Men, during your wife's pregnancy, you will be taking a back seat or more supportive role, but now is your opportunity to plant seeds of good health in the life of your future child.

*See Chapter 12*

Diet is important. A detoxification and cleansing program is a very good idea. Try to complete the program at least several months before conception. If there are any signs of yeast infection, both man and woman should try a yeast control program

> ## *Giving Your Child a Death Sentence*
>
> Smoking is fatal – both for the smoker and for those around him. This fact is undeniable and new evidence is coming out every day. Both parents should do whatever it takes to stop well before conception and take particular care in following a cleansing program. Pregnancy can be a stressful time both for the future mother and father. Since most smokers turn to cigarettes during times of stress, quitting becomes even more difficult. Besides, if you wait till you are pregnant to stop, damage will have already been done to the unborn child.

such as the one outlined in *Healthy Steps*. If one partner has yeast, it is very likely that the other one will have it as well, since yeast is easily passed during intimacy and intercourse. Severe cases of Candida Albicans yeast infection can result in infertility. Milder cases can be passed on to the child and show up in the form of allergies, thrush, skin rashes and respiratory difficulties.

There are also environmental concerns which should be considered. Exposure to pollution, strong chemicals and electro-magnetic radiation (EMR) may affect both fertility and health. If it is impossible to eliminate exposure, at least minimize it and take additional antioxidants.

Conception is a miracle of life. During intercourse, between 20 and 200 million sperm are released into the woman's vagina. If the conditions are right, one of those sperm will reach and fertilize the egg. If the egg and sperm are healthy and if the following guidelines are followed, approximately nine months later, a beautiful, healthy baby will look out at the world for the first time.

## Pregnancy

The first trimester (three months) of pregnancy is perhaps the most critical time in a baby's life. This is a period of incredibly

*The first trimester (three months) of pregnancy – the most critical time in a baby's life.*

rapid growth. The baby grows from one microscopic cell to a body three and a half inches (nine centimeters) long with fingers and toes, eyes, ears, mouth and nose.

During this time the baby is most susceptible to environmental hazards such as cigarette smoke, EMR, X-rays and chemical pollutants. It is also during this time that the baby is most sensitive to dietary indiscretions on the part of the mother. Substances like nicotine, alcohol, drugs and chemical food additives can interfere with the fetal enzyme system and inhibit growth factors. Therefore, by all means avoid alcohol, nicotine and caffeine. Do your best to stay away from drugs and foods with additives, preservatives and artificial colors and flavors.

Typically, the mother will feel fatigued both physically and emotionally. This should come as no surprise since the metabolic activity each day is approximately equal to that needed for climbing Mt. Everest. Do your best to get adequate rest. By all means, eat regularly and be sure your body is getting a steady and sufficient supply of nutrients. This will help ensure a smoother pregnancy for both mother and child.

Morning sickness is a common plague of many pregnant women. Unfortunately, the feelings of nausea and episodes of vomiting may strike at any time throughout the day. Additional intake of protein, the B vitamins and particularly B6 (up to 250 milligrams a day) may be helpful. Vitamin C and ginger can also provide some relief.

Good nutrition is vital throughout pregnancy. The developing fetus must get all of its nutrition from the food taken in by the mother. If there are deficiencies, some part of the development process may be negatively affected resulting in a stillbirth, a premature infant of low birth weight, a baby with brain damage (including "minor" things like impaired intelligence and psychological disturbances) or a baby with weakened immunity.

*Supplements for pregnancy.*

A number of nutrients are particularly important during

pregnancy and others may be helpful for childbirth.

Protein, calcium and iron are very important for the development of the bones, soft tissues and blood of the fetus. During pregnancy a woman's blood volume must increase by 20 percent, so protein and iron are very important for her as well. Vitamins C and K and the bioflavonoids are necessary to strengthen blood vessels and to prevent excessive bleeding.

*Now is the time to begin learning about breast feeding.*

See page 170. Many public libraries have helpful books and videos on technique. Practice relaxing.

---

### Common Pregnancy Problems

Edema – vitamin C, vitamin E, potassium -rich foods

Hemorrhaging – vitamin C with bioflavonoids, vitamin E (up to 200 IU with each meal), vitamin K

Itchy skin – aloe vera topically

Morning sickness – vitamin B6, vitamin C with bioflavanoids, vitamin K, ginger

Miscarriage, to prevent – vitamin C (500 milligrams to 4 grams increasing to as much as 10-15 grams by end of pregnancy) with bioflavonoids, folic acid

Muscle cramps – calcium, B vitamins (especially B6), magnesium

Restless legs – vitamin E

Stretch marks – vitamin E, zinc, aloe vera topically

Toxemia – (may be caused by poor nutrition or overuse of diuretics) good nutrition, magnesium, vitamin B6, choline, protein, vitamin E

---

## Smoother Labor and Delivery

Calcium is known to decrease pain. Taking 2000 milligrams between the beginning of labor and arrival at the hospital has helped many women. Zinc, protein, magnesium, potassium and essential fatty acids may also help. Vitamin E increases elasticity and expandability of vaginal muscles.

Raspberrry leaf tea has a rich history of preventing miscarriages and helping to make pregnancy and delivery easier. Many women like to drink a cup every day throughout their pregnancies. (Add one teaspoon dried leaves to one cup boiling water. Let steep for 15 minutes.)

However, it is as an aid to labor and delivery that raspberry leaf tea is most loved by women, particularly in Great Britain. When labor begins, pour two cups of boiling water over two tablespoons of tea leaves. Let steep for 30 minutes. Drink one cup as hot as possible. Be prepared to go to the hospital immediately. Better yet, go to the hospital and drink the tea in the parking lot. The other cup may be drunk in the delivery room.

Contractions and dilation may come on very quickly. You may even want to warn the hospital staff as they are often surprised.

After delivery, drinking raspberry leaf tea may help decrease uterine swelling and cut down on post partum bleeding.

# Chapter 15

# Special Concerns for Infants and Children

## by Ron Zehr

We can never underestimate how significant pregnancy and the first two years after birth are to a child's life. It could be said that before and during pregnancy, the foundation for the health of the child is being laid; during the first two years, the general framework is established.

### The First Year

For good health a newborn needs two things more than anything else: breast milk and love.

Discussing the importance of love and physical touching is outside of the scope of this book, but suffice it to say that a child's physical health and particularly mental and emotional health and development are greatly affected by the physical and personal expressions of love bestowed on her.

*A newborn needs two things more than anything else: breast milk and love.*

## The Perfect Food

A mother's breasts' have the amazing ability to produce milk with the precise nutrient content needed for an infant as he develops. Milk produced in the morning is slightly different from evening milk. As he grows, his needs change and so the makeup of the milk adjusts accordingly.

Breast milk is highly digestible and easy on the young digestive system. In fact, a breast-fed baby will tend to have fewer bowel movements because almost all of the milk will be used by the body. When they do come, the stools will tend to be smaller in volume and have an almost pleasant, sweet odor. (Hard to imagine, isn't it?) They will also be softer which will mean that the baby has to strain less and will have less problem with constipation.

*Breast milk is the perfect food for a newborn infant.*

Breast-fed babies also tend to have
- fewer ear infections,
- less problems with diaper rash (unless the mother has a yeast infection or has been eating sugar).
- fewer gastrointestinal infections
- fewer respiratory infections and
- stronger immune systems overall.

In general, they grow up to have
- higher IQs
- less incidence of diabetes
- less incidence of multiple sclerosis,
- fewer problems with allergies and
- better emotional and mental stability.

## A Nursing Mother's Diet

Poor nutrition while breast feeding tends to decrease the quantity of milk rather than the quality. The body will tend to draw from the mother's supply of nutrients. Of course, over the long run, the mother will become depleted, so good nutrition habits should always be practiced.

It is also important to be aware that whatever toxins or allergens the mother takes into her body will be passed on through the breast milk. Therefore, the ingestion of nicotine, caffeine, alcohol, drugs of any kind, food additives and preservatives may have a negative effect on the baby. Furthermore, the baby will have a much more difficult time handling these substances. Caffeine, for example, passes through most adults in about four hours, but takes up to 12 hours to pass through the system of an infant. A breast-fed baby whose mother drinks two cups of coffee a day could easily be on a constant 24-hour caffeine high.

*Caffeine is found in coffee, many teas, chocolate and colas.*

A baby may also be sensitive to certain foods eaten by the mother. Dairy products, citrus fruit, wheat and strawberries are among the most common offenders. Spicy foods may also cause problems if the mother has not been eating them on an ongoing basis. If they have been eaten during pregnancy, the nursing infant usually will not react to them.

Pure water is very important for a nursing mother who may be producing a number of cups of milk each day. Women who produce insufficient milk may be chronically dehydrated and simply increasing water consumption may solve the problem.

*Drink lots of water!*

## (Almost) Every Woman Can Nurse

Most women can nurse their newborn infants. In fact, even adoptive mothers have been known to stimulate milk production and breast-feed their adopted babies.

Probably the single most important technique to learn is to relax. There is only a small amount of milk at the front of the breast immediately behind the nipple. The baby will get this milk

*Practice relaxing.*

with the first few sucks. His appetite will be wetted and he will suck more. Regardless of how much he sucks, however, he will not get the rich "hind" milk unless the mother "lets down." In order for letdown to occur, the mother must be relaxed.

Milk production is a matter of supply and demand. Demand will vary depending on the growth patterns of the infant. If your baby seems to want to nurse constantly, don't assume that she is not getting enough or that you have run out of milk. She may be about to enter a growth spurt. Her more vigorous and frequent sucking is signalling your body to begin producing more milk.

*To get your baby started sucking, squeeze a little milk onto the nipple.*

The breast nipple is very different from any pacifier or bottle nipple and the sucking method varies accordingly. If at all possible, do not let your infant suck on a pacifier or bottle for the first four to six weeks. This will help avoid nipple confusion in which the infant forgets how to suck from the breast.

Once the sucking pattern has been firmly established, you can express milk manually or with one of the pumps on the market and store or freeze it for feeding times when you are away from your baby.

## Dealing with Breast Infections

Many mothers, especially first time nursers, get breast infections most often between the tenth and twenty-eighth day. The breast or part of the breast becomes red, sore and swollen. The infection may be accompanied by fever or chills.

Conventional medicine treats breast infections with antibiotics. Antibiotics can wreak havoc on the body at the best of times. For a nursing mother, they may cause even more problems. Not only do they encourage yeast infection in the mother, but also they affect the health of the baby. Often the yeast of the mother will be passed on to the baby and manifest itself in the form of thrush or diaper rash. The antibiotic, itself, will be passed

---

### Tips for Easier Nursing

- practice relaxing
- if possible, nurse in the same comfortable bed or chair
- guard against nipple confusion
- drink lots of liquids
- nurse from both breasts at each feeding
- elevate your feet to protect your back
- use the time to bond with your child

If you are having trouble, contact a lactation consultant or the local branch of La Leche League.

---

on to the baby as well. Babies frequently react with diarrhea and colic-like symptoms.

The best way to treat a breast infection is with rest, massage and cabbage leaves. Heat several cabbage leaves in boiling water until they are soft and pliable. Apply them as a hot compress over the affected area of the breast for 10 minutes. Do this every two to three hours, just before each breast-feeding session. You may want to put the cabbage leaves in a disposable diaper. It holds the heat well. Be careful not to burn yourself. Massage the sore area with your fingers and knuckles, focusing on any lumps you find. It will hurt. As you massage, try to express milk from the affected area.

Do not avoid breast-feeding. The milk moving through the ducts will help to clear up the infection. You may also want to take extra vitamin C, zinc and beta carotene. Within two to three days, you should be back to normal.

*If your infant cannot suck, but must be bottle fed, you can still express milk and give that to him rather than formula.*

## What if I Can't Breast Feed

A few women cannot breast-feed. Breast surgery occasionally severs some of the milk ducts. Sometimes, a mother must go on medication which could be dangerous if passed to the baby.

Sometimes, a baby cannot suck. If breast-feeding is not an option for you, or, if you simply choose not to, there are still things you can do to give your child a better chance at good health. Use the best formula available with purified water. With your doctor's supervision, you may want to try goat's milk with yogurt (see sections coming up on Weaning and Nutrition in the first year).

If your infant cannot suck, but must be bottle fed, you can still express milk and give that to him rather than formula. If you cannot breast-feed due to the medication you are on, express milk anyway and throw it out. This will keep your body producing so that when the medication is finished, you may still be able to nurse.

## Weaning

It is good if breast-feeding can continue as long as possible. Most of the studies which have shown the benefits of breast-feeding were with infants who were breast-fed exclusively for the first six months. This, of course, may be impossible, but try to get as close to six months as you can before introducing other foods. When you do it, be sure to proceed slowly. Introduce very small portions at a time.

*Honey – No! Babies under a year of age should not have honey because it may contain botulism spores.*

The best thing to begin weaning with is goat's milk and yogurt. Goats milk is sometimes called "orphan's milk" because in many cultures it is fed to all species of orphaned animals. It is far easier to digest and has a much better nutrient composition than cows milk. Try to get it unpasteurized if possible. Since it freezes well, you can buy it in quantity and store it in a deep freezer for up to six months.

Yogurt should be unflavored and unsweetened. It should contain live bacteria cultures. While you may want to try giving your infant yogurt on a spoon (no more than a teaspoon at a time to start), he may prefer the yogurt-goat's milk mix. Mix one-

> ### *What about Sweeteners?*
>
> Babies do not need sweeteners in their cereals. They are not born with a "sweet tooth" so why develop it. If you use any sweetener at all, try sorghum or blackstrap molasses. It contains relatively high amounts of minerals, particularly iron and calcium, and may even be a good addition to the diet of a six month old.

third cup of yogurt with two-thirds cups of goat's milk, then strain before putting it into a bottle. Go easy on the fruit juices. They are highly concentrated in fruit sugars. To give your infant extra liquid use purified water or dilute one part of pure (unsweetened) juice with about four or five parts of water (purified, of course). Avoid apple, citrus and berry juices in the early stages as they tend to be quite acidic. Apple can be introduced gradually; be careful with citrus juices until one or two years of age. Now is a great time to get your child into a habit of drinking lots of liquid each day. Frequently offer her the diluted juice or plain purified water.

This is also the time when you are "programing" your child's taste buds, so be alert to what you give her. To you, the diluted juice may taste too weak and the plain yogurt too tart. To her, they will taste just fine.

Once your child is five to six months old you can begin introducing "solid" food. However, you may wish to wait until the first birthday. Breast milk can meet all your baby's nutrient requirements until he is a year old. After that time, solid foods should definitely be added. In addition to yogurt, you can begin with grains. Rice cereal is a good place to start. Unfortunately, commercial brands often have additives or use white rice. You can buy brown rice (organic, if available) and easily grind it yourself in a mini grain/coffee grinder. Grind enough for several days and store it in the freezer so it does not go rancid.

When you are ready to prepare the cereal, mix one-third cup of the rice with two-thirds of a cup of hot water. Heat on the stove until bubbling, or until it thickens. This should give you enough for several days and it can be stored in the refrigerator. Depending on how long you cook the cereal, it may need to be thinned with a little milk (breast or goats) or yogurt. At first, your infant will probably only take a tablespoon or two at a time.

You may be surprised to observe that even though she is eating some solid food, your baby will still be wanting as much milk as before. The digestive system needs to adjust to food other than the highly digestible milk. It may take several weeks or even months until it can really assimilate the nutrients in the cereal, and you see a decrease in the volume of milk consumed.

## When to Stop Nursing

Continue nursing, if you can, even if it is only several times a day, until your child is one or even two years old. The Hunza people of the Himalayas are known to be the healthiest and longest living people on earth. They nurse their children until they are three years old. They also carefully space their children so each child can get all the breast milk available.

Recent research also suggests that about two years after delivery, a mother's milk contains a second surge of antibodies and other immune factors.

*Even if you need to work outside the home, you can still nurse morning and evening.*

Even if you need to work outside the home, you can still nurse morning and evening. Depending on your ability to relax and your work environment, you may be able to express milk during the day and bring the milk home for freezing or for use the next day. Expressed breast milk can be stored at room temperature for eight to ten hours as long as it is kept away from direst sunlight or heat sources. It will keep in the refrigerator for up to 72 hours. If you nurse or pump regularly, your body will have a supply available at the same time each day.

## Introducing Other Foods

As your baby becomes accustomed to the rice cereal, you can gradually introduce other whole grains. Again, organic is best, if possible. Try to stay away from wheat until at least one year as it may cause a reaction. Millet, oats, barley and quinoa are all good grains to add.

Introduce new foods one at a time. Wait at least four to five days before introducing another new food. This will allow you to immediately identify allergies. If you suspect an allergy, eliminate that food and try introducing it several months later when the child is older.

*Introduce new foods one at a time.*

Mashed or pureed vegetables and fruits may also be introduced at this time. Good ones to start with are sweet potatoes, peas, squash, baby lima beans, beets, carrots, turnips and broccoli. You can then follow with bananas, papayas and avocados.

You may be wondering, "What about commercial baby foods?" Most baby food manufacturers have finally stopped putting salt, sugar, artificial colors and other additives into their products. Unfortunately, many still over process the food and then add relatively large quantities of water.

Making your own baby food is a little more work, but many parents are convinced that the investment is worth the effort. Steam the vegetables first and then mash them. Hand grinders are available at many baby supply stores and are convenient and simple to use and clean. You may want to do up a week's worth of vegetables at a time. The mashed food can be frozen in ice cube trays for easy use later on.

## How Often Do I Feed?

Initially, you will only want to give your child one food at a time and probably only one meal per day. After a few months, begin to combine two foods, and feed two meals. By about ten months your child can be eating three meals a day plus finger food snacks. You may be only breast-feeding (or giving the yogurt-goat's milk mixture) twice a day.

*The key to diet is variety.*

The key to diet is variety. This will help to prevent allergies from developing and will also acquaint your child's taste buds with many different foods.

## Nutrition for Children

As you introduce foods to your young child, you are setting eating habits that may stay with her for life. Be careful what you give her, and be careful what example you set. In general, the principles described elsewhere in this book also apply to children. Because children usually have faster metabolisms, they may need to eat more frequently and may need something more substantial in the mornings.

*As much as possible, avoid food additives.*

As much as possible, avoid food additives. Avoid sugar. It is found in too many foods designed for children. Practice label reading and learn to recognize sugar by other names. Be careful of cookies, cakes, crackers, cereals and juices.

There are many cookbooks with recipes for sugar-free cakes and cookies. Most healthfood stores also have a selection. You may pay more, but remember it is a wise investment.

### Fruit

*Fresh fruit is a great snack food.*

Fresh fruit is a great snack food. With very young children, of course, be careful of choking hazards. Initially, all fruit should be pureed. Later, soft fruits can be cut into small bite-sized pieces and hard fruits can be grated. Always grate apples or cut them into thin slices. Cut grapes and larger berries in half. Kiwi is another fruit that children often love – if they haven't been spoiled with sugary snacks. Try to give your child at least three servings of fruit a day.

In the winter, fresh fruit may be hard to obtain, but you can also thaw frozen fruit and mix it with cereal or yogurt. Avoid canned fruit as it often contains sugar and tends to have fewer nutrients left in it.

## Vegetables

A variety of vegetables should be served at least twice a day. Don't forget to include dark-leafed plants. If you feed the child a variety as an infant, they are more likely to be less fussy later on.

## Protein

There is increasing concern among many nutritionists over feeding meat to children. There is some evidence that children cannot handle it until they are at least four years old and some feel that it is wise to wait until a child is even older (7-12). Not only do young children have difficulty getting value from it, but the meat can lead to health problems over the long run. When and if you do choose to introduce it, do so in very small portions.

*There is increasing concern among many nutritionists over feeding meat to children.*

Children need protein. Protein, however, can be obtained from many sources.

- Legumes can be cooked and pureed,
- Nut butters can be mixed with cereals for infants or put on bread for older children (Avoid peanuts until the child is at least two years old, since they are frequent allergens.),
- Cottage cheese and yogurt (with live bacteria cultures) are easy to digest,
- Cheese and cream cheese in moderation,
- Tofu, soya cheese or soya burgers and hotdogs (cut them lengthwise and into small pieces to eliminate choking hazard),
- Goat's milk,
- Whole grains and spirulina.

*Protein sources*

### Grains

Whole grains are an excellent source of energy and nutrients and can be fed to children in many forms. Children love bread and noodles. Be sure to buy whole grain varieties. If they are a frequent part of your menu, vary the grains.

## Dealing with a Fussy Eater

*Suggested snacks:*
- *fruit*
- *vegetables (lightly cooked for toddlers)*
- *rice cakes*
- *popsicles from unsweetened fruit juices*
- *bread (wholegrain)*
- *nut butters (avoid peanuts)*
- *cheese*

Most battles over food are really not about food, but about control, dominance. Who will be king? (or queen?) Yes, that little bundle of joy is defying your authority and proclaiming to all, "I can decide myself what I am going to eat! And no one can make me change my mind!"

When this happens, you have several options:

• Rise to the challenge. Issue a decree that you have no hope of ever enforcing. "You are NOT getting out of your high chair until you have eaten every bite."

Two hours later, your nerves are frazzled. The child is either wailing or sitting there stone-faced in icy silence. The bowl may still be full or it may be empty with food strewn across the floor, or the dog may be gratefully licking his chops.

You lift the child from the high chair, mumbling as you do it, "Don't think that I'm going to let you off so easily next time." Your child knows better. "Another victory. Yes!" she thinks to herself.

• Use a cannon. No, not literally. Force the child's mouth open. Threaten punishment worthy of a heinous crime. Don't give in regardless how much he screams. In fear for his life, your child may actually swallow that little mouthful. You may end up with either a broken child or miserable mealtimes.

• Use intelligence and tactical maneuvering greater than what your toddler is capable of. Offer a reward if she eats one, two or three bites of the offensive food. The reward could be food or it could be a horsey ride, a favorite story, a game or some other social treat. The reward need not be grandiose. Whatever you do, do not give the reward unless she meets the requirement, and do not change the requirement.

Try the "one-bite-one-bite" tactic – a bite of the offending food followed by a bite of a yummy food.

If nothing seems to work, end the meal. Chances are good that tomorrow or the next day your child will have moved onto other battles and eat that "offensive" food without a second thought.

If the negative reaction is constant, it could indicate an allergy. If you suspect this, avoid the offending food for a few months, then test it.

## Dealing with Sickness

Practicing good health care means that sickness need not be a frequent occurrence. However, it will happen. When it does, practice what has been presented elsewhere in this book. Remember that even the body of a young child has the ability to heal itself.

*Practicing good health care means that sickness need not be a frequent occurrence.*

The average toddler or young child gets about 12 colds a year. If you are following what has been laid out in this chapter, your child should get fewer than that, but colds and flu will probably pay visits nonetheless.

### Antibiotics

It is appalling how frequently antibiotics are given to many young children. Use natural remedies unless the problem is serious. Vitamin C and aloe vera can be given even to young infants. Some herbs can also be given.

If you must give your child antibiotics, be sure to also give additional yogurt or acidophilus to help replenish the good bacteria which are killed by the antibiotics.

### Colic

The exact cause of colic is not known, although some things seem to aggravate it. Immediate relief can sometimes be obtained by using a few drops of an herbal remedy for gastrointestinal upsets. Some parents have also given their infants pure aloe vera juice. (Be sure to strain out any pulp.) Some parents have also found that massaging the abdomen very gently may also bring relief.

While you may be able to get through the immediate episode by using the methods described above, prevention really is the key. Consider carefully the diet of the nursing mother and eliminate any suspect foods. Dairy products are common offenders. Citrus fruit may also cause irritation.

Generally, foods will take about four to eight hours to get into the breast milk. Consider what you ate approximately that long before the last feeding. If there was anything unusual, don't eat it again for a few days; then try it and observe the reaction in your baby.

*Fever is a sign that the body is marshalling its forces to fight against infection.*

### Fever

It really is a scary thing when your child lies in your arms, hot and feverish. The natural tendency is to do whatever we can to make him "feel better." Unfortunately, our attempts may often frustrate the body's natural healing process.

Fever is a sign that the body is marshalling its forces to fight against infection. Normally, a healthy child is well able to overcome whatever virus or bacteria he is fighting.

Pediatrician Robert S. Mendelsohn, M.D., says that more important than the height of a child's temperature is the overall appearance, behavior and attitude of the child. He suggests that if the child appears extremely "listless or confused or displays other disturbingly abnormal behavior, a call to your doctor may be warranted if the symptoms persist for a day or two."

The exception is with very young infants. During the delivery process, a newborn may contact infections in a number of ways. If fever develops as a result, it is best to see a doctor.


## Vaccinations

For over 50 years, vaccinations have been unquestioningly accepted by loving, yet uninformed parents. We've been told that they are necessary, and that they are perfectly safe. Neither may be the case.

*Vaccination Considerations*

Vaccination may not be any help at all in protecting against disease. Consider the following:

• There is no convincing scientific evidence that mass immunization programs are effective. Incidents of most of the diseases commonly vaccinated against were declining before the programs were introduced. As these diseases diminished or disappeared in the USA, they disappeared simultaneously in Europe where mass immunization did not take place.

• Most of the diseases vaccinated against are relatively harmless to children but can have serious consequences for adults. Some of the vaccines appear to wear out and leave adults vulnerable. In addition, vaccine-resistant strains of some of these diseases are developing with adults falling victim most often.

*Long term effects*

• Most cases of polio, measles and rubella (German measles) occur in vaccinated adults and children. When Germany and France began vaccinating against diphtheria, the number of cases of the disease skyrocketed.

Furthermore vaccinations may be dangerous to the health of your child.

*Could be danger-*
*ous!*

• The measles and whooping cough (pertussis) vaccines may cause seizures, brain damage and death.

• The rubella vaccine may cause high fever, inner ear damage, anaphylactic shock and loss of consciousness.

• The mumps vaccine may cause rashes, itching, febrile seizures and nerve deafness.

• The diphtheria, pertussis and tetanus (DPT) vaccine may be a factor in sudden infant death syndrome (SIDS). A University of Nevada Medical School found that of 103 babies who died of SIDS, 70 percent had been vaccinated with DPT within three weeks of death. SIDS frequencies have peak occurrences immediately following the primary doses of DPT at two, four and six months of age.

• In less than two years time, $82 million was awarded as compensation in the United States alone for deaths and injuries from vaccinations.

• Autism occurred in the United States, Japan and Europe at the same time as the introduction of the pertussis vaccine.

• Long-term effects are unknown, but some scientists suspect vaccinations may be a factor in the rise of autoimmune and immune deficiency diseases.

The decision of whether or not to vaccinate is a difficult one and should not be made lightly. Sadly, most of the information distributed by doctors and health workers is intended to convince not inform. So convinced has our society become that many parents are regarded almost as child abusers when they refuse to submit their children to what they see as an unproven and dangerous procedure.

The decision must be yours. Consider it carefully, but by all means get all of the facts.

# Chapter 16

# The Spiritual Dimension of Man

While the focus of this book is physical health, we all realize that there is much more to life than having a healthy physical body. The spiritual dimension of man is generally regarded as an important factor in wholeness and necessary for man's total fulfillment. However, since the topic is also a potential source of controversy, it is generally avoided, or, if presented, is too often done in a dogmatic and sometimes offensive way. In this chapter I will venture into this matter, because for me personally and in my life's observations it has tremendous significance.

Before I proceed, I will state that my personal stance is Christian. This means that I have accepted Jesus Christ as the center and focus of my life, and the Bible as my ultimate authority. I desire daily to please Him, and although at times I fail, I find Him forgiving, and so my relationship with Him has grown closer over more than forty years of knowing and walking with Him. I declare this so that the reader will know that I am not trying to hide anything or to push something on the reader

*There is much more to life than having a healthy physical body.*

against his will. If this perspective is unacceptable to you, please feel free to use the balance of this book to whatever extent you find it helpful. Even if you feel that this perspective is not for you, reading this chapter may help you to better understand how I and others perceive spiritual things.

## Three Parts of Man

*To be complete and fulfilled, we must be healthy in body, soul and spirit.*

It is helpful for our discussion to consider man as a being of three parts: body, soul, and spirit. To be complete and fulfilled, we must be healthy in body, soul and spirit. I am, of course, aware that there is considerable overlap in these areas, but to help us to perceive the uniqueness of each, please allow me to separate them for the purpose of this discussion.

### The Body

The outward and most obvious part of man is the body. It is the visible, tangible and physical aspect made up of flesh, blood and bones. It might be considered the "house" that the soul and spirit inhabit. The body, being physical, relates to the physical realm around it. Its faculties convey to us touch, sights, sounds, tastes and odors. In this way it can substantiate and allow us to relate to the physical world.

*The body is the "house" that the soul and spirit inhabit.*

If our body is injured, we experience physical pain. The body's health is dependent on proper food, rest and protection. The health of the body is so crucial because it is the "house" or vehicle in which our soul and spirit dwell and in which they are conveyed while here on earth. On the other hand, if we were merely a body, we would in effect be simply a "vegetable" without thought or feeling. As important and amazing as our body is, it is yet secondary and simple in comparison to our soul and spirit!

### The Soul

Man, of course, is also a psychological being. Our soul,

consisting of our mind, our emotions and our will must also be healthy in order for us to live with meaning and enjoyment. Though not physically tangible like the body, our soul is, nevertheless, equally real.

Consider the matter of pain. A physical object such as a stick can cause pain to my body which is the physical part of my being. However, my soul can experience pain from something that is very real yet not physical. A verbal criticism, a misunderstanding or psychological abuse all cause this kind of pain.

A psychologist or psychiatrist studies and seeks to help people function and be healthy in the realm of the soul. Since that is not our intent here, we wish merely to affirm the premise that the soul may be seen as a distinct part of the human person. It may also be considered to function in and relate to psychological things in the psychological realm.

### The Spirit

Does man have a spirit? Is there a spiritual realm? How do we know or how do we contact this realm? These and other similar questions have been asked by all serious minded persons since the beginning of time. It seems to me that the intense interest of man concerning this matter suggests at least a strong probability that there is such a realm – a spiritual realm to be realized and enjoyed, a realm so crucial to the existence of man that the meaning and purpose of human life cannot be fully realized apart from having a healthy spiritual dimension. Someone has suggested, "There does seem to be a God-shaped vacuum in man, and until it is filled, man cannot have complete inner rest."

I realize that many take the view that this is a highly personal matter, and that each person must find the answer for herself. I have found this true in the sense that we must each personally take initiative to discover the answer which is available and waiting for us to accept. It is not true, however, if we, in effect, assume that we can each create our own answer to suit our own

*Our soul, though not physically tangible like the body, is, nevertheless, equally real.*

*There does seem to be a God-shaped vacuum in man.*

inclination. If there is a spiritual realm, then it existed before I did, and it originated with Someone far beyond me, so I had best humble myself to seek in an asking way, rather than in a presumptuous way.

The God whom I have come to know hears and answers the humble, whereas the arrogant are left to their own devices. Since this God is Spirit, He can be known only as we allow Him to disclose Himself to our spirit in His way. I am not interested in creating my own god from my thought or ingenuity. I would rather ask the God who created me to reveal Himself to me.

*He can be known only as we allow Him to disclose Himself to our spirit in His way.*

Please allow me to explain what I perceive to be the Biblical answer to this dilemma – an answer that gives my life deep present joy, as well as permanent and eternal meaning and purpose. I consider it not as self discovery, but a wonderful undeserved gift for which I shall be eternally grateful. I find it impossible to share this matter without referring to the Bible, since it is my exclusive resource on the matter. A primary reason that I accept the Bible totally is because it speaks to and clarifies the deep inner sense of my "heart of hearts" (i.e. my spirit).

For those wishing to check these matters out personally, let me simply cite a few references to biblically establish the existence of man's spirit. Job 32:8; Psalms 31:5; 143:4; Proverbs 16:2; Ezekiel 11:19; Matthew 26:41; John 4:24; 1 Corinthians 2:11; 1 Thessalonians 5:23; Hebrews 4:12.

### The History of Man's Spirit

Now let's take a brief look at the history of man's spirit as revealed in the Bible. According to Genesis, the first book of the Bible, God, Who is Spirit, created man as body, soul, and spirit intending to have an intimate spiritual relationship with man via man's spirit. God chose to allow man to exercise a free will and to choose between two options. Man could choose to eat of the Tree of Life which symbolized the spiritual Life of God. This would place man in dependence, in harmony and in fellowship with God. This Life would enliven man's spirit making spiritual communication continuously possible.

The other option was symbolized by the Tree of the Knowledge of Good and Evil. God had already told man that choosing this option would put him under a sentence of death. This choice would indicate a determination by man to be independent from God, self-reliant and self-centered. The latter choice had already been taken by a leading angel, Satan, who had rebelled against God and become alienated from him. Satan appeared, in the form of a serpent, to strongly influence man to choose independence from God, which would unwittingly mean submission to Satan's own influence. Man accepted the influence of Satan, God's enemy, and ate of the Tree of the Knowledge of Good and Evil. This is referred to as the "fall of man." This is why there is evil, also referred to as "sin," in the basic nature of human beings.

The resulting sinful condition caused two problems: alienation and death. Since God is sinless and holy, there was an immediate alienation or separation between God and man. Man became fearful, distrusting and suspicious of God, and filled with questions toward God. We will call this first problem, alienation.

The second problem is that at the moment of man's sin, something within man ceased functioning, or died. That which died was man's spirit. Consequently, the part of man's being which could substantiate or relate to the spiritual realm became inoperative. From that time on, man could only use his soul to imagine, speculate and theorize about spiritual matters. Anyone engaging the "fallen" mind to perceive God will, of course, end up with a creation of his own imagination, always somewhat different from anyone else's idea.

Surprisingly, even in spite of man's alienated condition, God was able to communicate with man in varying degrees, but always in a limited way.

*God chose to allow man to exercise a free will and to choose between two options.*

*The Tree of Life
or
the Tree of Knowledge
of Good and Evil?*

_____ *Part Two*
*Good Health as a Daily Practice*

In the first part of the Bible, God implies that in the future He would find a way to reach man and carry out His original intention. At times He communicated quite specifically through certain persons. In retrospect, we see that these persons were prototypes, or prior models, of the real person whom God would eventually send to resolve man's dilemma. In fact, everything in the first half of the Bible seems to be pointing toward a certain time, place and person.

## The Answer to the Dilemma

Eventually, the answer came in the person of Jesus Christ. He was not born sinful. He lived a sinless life and He was alive in His spirit and in communication with God His Father. Since Jesus was sinless, He did not deserve to die, so He was able to die on behalf of those who were guilty and under the sentence of death, a death which had already affected them. When Jesus was crucified and died, He offered his life voluntarily to God in the place of everyone who was under the sentence of death.

*Eventually, the answer to man's dilemma came.*

This pardon is now available to anyone who will acknowledge their own guilt and accept Christ's death on their behalf. Anyone who does this is thereby able to resolve the first problem, that of alienation. Because God has declared that he who accepts the death of Christ on their behalf can be reconciled to or made right with Him, God can now accept and freely relate to all those who accept this offer.

While Christ's death was able to resolve the problem of alienation, what about the problem of spiritual death? This problem required not death, but life, even resurrected life! Three days after His death, Christ arose! That's what Easter is all about. After He resurrected, He was made to be what the Bible calls a "life-giving spirit," able to impart spiritual life into those who accept Him. He continues this activity in the form of the Holy Spirit. Receiving this new life, sometimes referred to as being born again, overcomes the second problem, spiritual death. Paul, a New Testament writer, describes his personal experience of having once been dead and then being made alive. Jesus, in reference to this experience, once told an older man called Nicodemus, "You must be born again."

*Now He is able to impart spiritual life into those who accept Him.*

Once the spirit of the believer has been made alive, it allows him suddenly to perceive and substantiate experiences and information which he was unable to realize before. Through the enlivened faculties of his spirit, he can receive information, sometimes referred to as revelation, which he was not able to perceive earlier merely by his body or soul. The writer Paul also declares that the soul or the human mind in itself cannot understand the things of the spirit; in fact they are foolishness to him. This is why a new believer is often regarded as so strange or so different from what he was before this new life experience, since a deep and permanent change has actually taken place.

This awakening to the spiritual realm is available to anyone through repentance from their sin, acceptance of the death of Christ on their behalf, and an opening of the heart to His new life. It is available to absolutely anyone, just for the asking. This is the "amazing grace" that inspired one of the most widely known songs in all of history. This song, *Amazing Grace,* was written by John Newton, formerly a violent and lawless slave trader, after he fell on his knees and took this offer. He described the effect of this new life with these words, "I once was lost, but now am found, was blind but now I see." Just before his death at age 82, he said, "I still marvel at this amazing grace!"

*The awakening to this spiritual realm is available to anyone.*

## The Growth of this New Life

I want to continue briefly to discuss how, after receiving this life, we can keep it dynamic and healthy. Like a physical birth, so the new birth is only a beginning. In both cases, the life received has inherent within itself a new nature. However, there is a crucial need for nourishment both for sustenance and growth, so that the life may be healthy, and realize its full potential. Just as food, exercise and social contact is necessary for our physical and psychological life, so our spiritual life has its needs.

The healthy growth of the spiritual life requires "spiritual" food and the exercise of our spirit. Some, even though they have been made alive spiritually, neither feed nor care for their spiritual life, so they are spiritually weak and sickly, or see little spiritual growth, and are like a neglected, malnourished infant.

For spiritual health, the primary, spiritual food must be reading and absorbing the Bible, God's Word. This will not only provide spiritual direction, but also nourishment for growth that we might mature and be strengthened in faith. Spiritual exercise involves prayer, study, fellowship with others, singing and responding to the leading of God's Spirit who lives in every real believer. Gradually, this develops an ever closer and deeper relationship with God, including a deep joy and warm inner peace, and an increasing evidence of the likeness of Christ in our lives. All this can be experienced here and now. In addition, the believer can have a solid assurance of an eternity in the presence of God with all those who have accepted His unmerited and unconditional offer of eternal life.

This all becomes very meaningful and exciting. But, since the subject of this book is physical health, I had better keep myself from getting too carried away. To those who strongly disagree with the above or have no interest in such matters, I thank you for your kind forbearance. With those who have a strong interest in these matters or desire more information, I would be delighted to share more, either in person or in writing. It is really true, God loves us and desires the very best for us. He will receive and bless all those who sincerely seek Him!

*Part Two* _____
*Good Health as a Daily Practice*

# PART THREE

# HEALTH PROBLEMS AND NATURAL REMEDIES

*Part Three*_____
*Health Problems and Natural Remedies*

# Chapter 17

# *Body Talk*

As we have lost the sense of personal responsibility for our own health, we have also lost a clear sense of our body. Our body has become like a machine to us. We use it for our purposes with little sensitivity to its needs. We supply just enough fuel and maintenance to keep it running, but keep a detached and rather impersonal attitude towards it.

In my lectures I often refer to the concept of hearing our body talking, and responding to its requests and directives. Inevitably, when I broach the topic, I see some eyebrows being raised. I can read the thoughts churning in some suspicious minds. "Where is this guy coming from? This sounds far-out, even a little spacey."

At that point I like to ask a frown-faced listener, "Does your body not speak to you?"

"I doubt it. I really don't get into that realm" is a typical response.

"Have you gone to the toilet today; have you eaten or slept lately?" I ask.

"Of course, doesn't everyone?" comes the skeptical reply.

"But why, or how did you know when to do these things?" I ask.

As the light slowly dawns, the reply comes, "I guess my body told me."

To press the point home, I then ask, "So your body does communicate, but what makes you think that all it can say is potty, yum-yum and night-night? You learned that by age three. Haven't you realized that your body wants to communicate beyond this elementary level?"

By this time in my lecture, the case for "body talk" is established, and we can develop the matter somewhat further.

## General Body Talk

In earlier sections of this book, we talked about food allergy testing. We also covered the matter of responding to our body's reaction to food, both in content and quantity. We pointed out how we are controlled by taste rather than the body's deeper indications which inform us of its real needs. These examples focus on the area we refer to here as body talk. Let's review them briefly, and then go on to see more ways that we can read our body's desire to communicate.

*Checking out allergic reactions.*

An allergic reaction occurs when our body's immune system perceives some element such as a bacteria, virus or toxin to be potentially harmful. It then launches a counterattack which may evoke a fever, puffy eyes, runny nose, etc. This reaction is certainly the body talking. The question should be "what is the body reacting to and why?" If it is a food allergy, the reaction could be to any number of the various foods being ingested.

The only sure way to really get the message is to avoid specific foods for at least five days and then reintroduce them one at a time. This way of isolating specific foods allows you to receive a clear message, because the reaction can be pinned down to a particular food. If our suspicion is correct, then when we avoid that food, the reaction should no longer occur. I share this example of screening for foods that cause allergic reactions because it illustrates one aspect of what I call body talk.

Our body could be quite instructive concerning what and how much we should eat. However, this capability tends to be overridden and frustrated starting in early childhood. For example, anything that has a sweet taste is described as "good." Many of us were taught always to finish everything on our plate. While this advice was well intentioned, its subtle result was to teach us to overeat! As children we heard statements such as "No dessert until you finish your meal." Of course, tradition has taught us that a meal is not complete without dessert. We were also conditioned to see desserts or sweets as a way of rewarding ourselves.

Now, when we indulge, we feel we deserve it, because we completed something difficult and therefore may reward ourselves by eating those chocolates.

With such programming, is it any wonder that our body's digestive system is in chaos and that there is very little chance of us hearing our body talk? If we could retune our hearing, what might we hear our body say concerning our eating? Here are some of the phrases we would probably hear it say: "that's enough, thanks; please stop; I can't handle that sugar now; I need hours to digest what I have, before I can properly handle more."

*Retune hearing to hear body talk.*

How often have you felt quite comfortable after eating a nice dinner? Unable to resist the pressure, for whatever reason, you eat pie and ice cream or other dessert. Soon after you feel heavy and sluggish, begin to belch and experience bloating and gas. This is body talk, but still, it seems, we don't get the message.

_____ *Part Three*
*Health Problems and Natural Remedies*

The classic breakfast of eggs, bacon, hash browns and butter soaked toast is a sickening blow to a body that has just awakened and is ready to eliminate its accumulated toxic waste. No wonder so many people need half the day to get going! Much more compatible would be a cup of hot water, some fruit, and perhaps some fiber. Try it for a week and see how much happier your body will be.

If we are willing to make some observations, we will begin to recognize what foods, eating times, and quantities will provide our body with maximum satisfaction and lead to its best performance. The same is true of learning how much rest our body needs.

*Listen to your body now, before it screams at you later!*

## Deeper Observations

I believe that we can even "hear" and learn what supplements our bodies are asking for. Personally, for years I have been on a fairly consistent supplement program. In addition to the basics, I find that for me, vitamin C is crucial for my body to maintain optimal performance, and the amount needed varies significantly. Under normal circumstances, about 1000 milligrams of vitamin C per day are adequate. When I travel over time zones and lecture night after night, I need about 3000 milligrams per day. If while I travel I get a raspy throat, or sense that I'm in a "pre-cold" mode, I take 4000-6000 milligrams per day. With this awareness and practice, after nearly twenty years and hundreds of tours, I have never had to miss one lecture, and have averaged less than one cold per year.

Sleep and good rest are another area where we too often ignore what our bodies are telling us. Even while I was a child, my mother observed that my good health was very much contingent on getting enough sleep. She used to say that when most children get sick they may need to see a doctor, but when

Albert gets sick he needs to sleep. When I didn't get enough sleep, I would become nauseous, have cramps and begin to vomit. If she would put me to bed, I would sleep twelve hours and be fine. For the first thirty years of my life, I tried everything conceivable to need less sleep, but with little success. To a lesser degree, this condition remains. Others may brag and boast that four, five or even six hours of sleep are all they need; my body says, "give me seven to eight and I'll serve you well, but give me less and I'll complain."

*The body is attempting to transmit a message.*

Accepting these "requests" and responding to my body has given me almost sixty healthy, trouble-free years, and I anticipate many more. I have come to conclude that if you listen and take care of your body, it will take care of you.

## Symptom Interpretation

Another area of body talk is learning to recognize and interpret symptoms. A headache, rash, swelling, itching, nausea, pain, redness, bloating, etc., are all attempts by the body to transmit a message.

If we apply the body talk concept, we will not merely settle for some medication to suppress the symptoms, but will take the time and effort to interpret and respond to what our body is trying to tell us.

## A Further Step in Listening to Our Bodies

My telephone rings. "Dr. Zehr, I was taking three vitamin C and then my friend said I should be taking four. What do you say?"

Someone sits across the desk from me. "Dr. Zehr, I am taking four alfalfa tablets, but I heard I should be taking six. Please tell me, what is the right amount?"

I reply, "Why don't you take a dozen and see what happens?"

"But how will I know if I am taking too much?"

"When you take too much alfalfa, you will start saying, 'moo' in your sleep!"

I share the above to illustrate a number of points. With the constant administration of potentially lethal medications all around us, we have been programed to believe that the exact amount is very crucial. Because of this, we have become focused on the prescription of experts, but oblivious to the indications of our body.

*Guidelines may be helpful, but learn to listen to your body.*

While certain guidelines may be helpful, in a sense, the amount of supplements one should take is rather a personal and subjective matter. Often my response to the question, "How much?" is rather general, like "Try two to four, and see how your body reacts." I say this deliberately to steer the person away from dependency on me, and towards hearing his body speaking.

Many nutritional counselors employ a technique referred to as bio-kinesiology, or muscle testing. The person being tested stands with her arm straight out from her body and resists the pressure that the tester will apply. The tester applies pressure to see how much resistance there is. Then a supplement or other element is held in the person's other hand and is placed against the stomach area. If at that point the extended arm is stronger, the item being tested is considered of positive value. If the person's arm is weaker, then the item being tested is considered of negative value.

The above method is really a form of listening to the body talk. With practice and sensitivity, I believe that each of us can learn to read our own body's responses and help ourselves and others.

# Chapter 18

# *Understanding Disease Categories*

A central premise of help yourself health care is to move beyond an attempt to merely deal with symptoms. While symptomatic relief may give us some immediate satisfaction, by now we have come to realize that real and permanent wellness requires that we address the cause. A certain underlying health frustration may well express itself in numerous symptoms. If we just chase the symptoms without altering the underlying cause, we will merely be rearranging symptoms.

As we have seen already, most health breakdown is a result of various factors, particularly inadequate supply, elimination and defence. Between these factors and particular diseases, there are also usually some general problems. These problems set up a particular situation where certain disease can be easily manifest.

For example, living in Vancouver, British Columbia, we have a moist and moderate climate with little severe cold in the winter. This sets up a situation where moss easily grows, especially in the shade. In other words, we might say that uncontrolled moss overgrowth is a symptom of a lack of sunlight combined with cool, moist conditions. We have found, however, that instead of trying to kill the moss, if we reduce the shade by clearing overhead branches, the moss is much less of a problem and often dies off on its own.

I have found that the following underlying conditions tend to make the body much more susceptible to certain diseases. If these conditions are recognized and altered where possible, many symptoms and even diseases can be overcome. This often makes it unnecessary to directly attack the disease, because now the body is able to do its own self-healing. This is like removing the nail in the shoe, instead of constantly trying to find new ways to heal the sore.

This is so significant that in our suggestions for dealing with the diseases listed in the next chapter, we will always recommend beginning with consideration of possible disease categories. With many diseases, if we adjust the conditions, the body will be able to recover from the disease on its own.

## Genetic – GN

*Be extra vigilant to overcome genetic weaknesses.*

This refers to conditions which have been inherited from one's parents. It may be a weakened or defective organ or system, such as a weak heart, kidneys or a nervous disorder. If it is simply a constitutional weakness, extra care and support for the weakened area may prevent breakdown. The concept that "I will have arthritis because my mother and grandmother had it" must be challenged. Rather, I should determine to be extra vigilant so that my body will be able to overcome this genetic weakness and overcome the potential problem. Under adverse conditions, including neglect, my body may begin to break down in these weaker areas. With a little extra care for the weaker member and good health management, I should be able to avoid such a breakdown.

In other cases, where a person is born with an inherent disability or incomplete function, we must find ways to adapt. Many times, the body has remarkable ways to compensate for loss or shortage. For instance, if one gland is weak or non-functioning, the other glands may make up for the shortage to a remarkable degree – if they are well supplied and cared for. Life is resilient and ingenious. Don't resign to a life of poor health just because of a genetic weakness. Give the rest of your body a little extra care and supply, and you will be pleasantly surprised at the health and vitality which can still be yours.

## Allergy or Immune Related – AIR

The immune system is amazing in its ability to defend and protect the human body. In order to accomplish this, it must preform meticulous surveillance over every minute element that contacts or enters the body. Any potentially harmful or un-friendly element must be identified, attacked and discarded at all costs. Sometimes this battle is furious, generating an elevated temperature and a temporary neglect of other important aspects of the body's needs.

With all of this constant bombardment, the immune system may become "skittish" and begin to suspect and reject otherwise normal and acceptable elements. At such a time, we conclude that the host has become "allergic" to whatever the offending element might be. The introduction of such allergens may easily preoccupy the immune system so that it neglects or becomes unable to properly maintain its general protection of the body. The areas neglected, often genetically weak areas, begin to develop problems and become the focus of medical attention. As these neglected areas break down (with symptoms such as skin disease, intestinal disorders or joint pain), each is addressed medically, often with little success.

*Allergens may "preoccupy" the immune system.*

If at such times, the allergy problem which set up the situation were addressed, then the body could enact its own recovery from the secondary breakdown. Employ the method described elsewhere to see if you can determine the offending allergen. When it is identified and removed, often the apparently "incurable" symptom begins to subside. The body is now able to relax from its frenzied attempt to fight the symptom, and get back to its real job of maintaining normal good health.

*For tips on allergy testing see 109 and 196.*

## Yeast or Infection Related – YIR

Very similar to the above allergy-related type of diseases is the problem of yeast or infection related conditions. The human body, especially the large intestine, carries a certain amount of yeast activity. An especially aggressive form which thrives on sugars is known as Candida Albicans. The friendly bacteria in the colon help to keep yeast in check. When antibiotics destroy the friendly bacteria, or a diet high in sugar feeds the yeast, it may grow rampantly and spread throughout the system.

The yeast overgrowth seems to choke and frustrate the body's vitality, and indirectly causes symptoms to flare up. Skin problems, such as acne, shingles, psoriasis and hives, as well as earaches may be indications of yeast overgrowth. Since it also invades the soft tissues of the vagina and bronchials, vaginal and respiratory problems also often result from yeast infections.

*For more on yeast infections, see **Healthy Steps.***

From the above, it is clear that treating a respiratory infection with antibiotics can easily become counterproductive. The antibiotics frustrate the immune system and kill the friendly bacteria giving the yeast more freedom to thrive, so it can rally for another attack on the bronchials. The same is true of ear infections and most skin problems. If natural antibiotics such as garlic or golden seal were used instead, and the yeast were brought under control, the immune system could be strengthened, and natural and permanent relief attained.

## Thyroid and Metabolism Related – TMR

The thyroid gland, located in the throat area, produces a number of different hormones of which thyroxine is the primary one. The amount of oxygen consumed by the body's cells and the rate of metabolism are both controlled by the thyroid. We might say that it sets the "idling speed" of the whole body.

Thyroid disorder is considered by some experts to be a classical phantom disease which secretly afflicts millions of people. While the thyroid gland is very hidden and grossly under recognized, its activity sends ripple effects throughout the entire body, and problems with the thyroid may well lie at the root of numerous health frustrations, both physical and mental.

*Thyroid disorder may be a phantom disease – secretly afflicting millions.*

*Hyperthyroidism,* also known as Graves disease, is a condition where the thyroid develops an overactive state. Usual symptoms are nervousness, intolerance for heat, rapid heartbeat, weight loss, tiredness, increased appetite, excessive thirst, difficult breathing, weak muscles, frequent urination and diarrhea. We could describe this as the body running too fast, or being hyper!

Studies published in May 1997 issue of *Townsend Letter for Doctors and Patients* report an apparent linkage between hyperthyroidism and aspartame consumption.

Multivitamin and mineral supplements, high B-Complex dosages, vitamins C and E and iodine can all help balance thyroid function. Broccoli, brussels sprouts, cabbage, kale, spinach, soybeans, peaches and pears can slow thyroid activity. Avoid caffeine, alcohol and soft drinks. Radioactive iodine is often advised, but be aware that it can have severe side effects.

*Hypothyroidism* is a much more common condition in which the thyroid gland secretes less than the normal amount of thyroxine. Heartbeat and breathing tend to be slower and heart action becomes weaker. Susceptibility to infection increases and body temperature is below normal. The patient may feel chilly, and the skin may be puffy, rough and thickened. Symptoms may include fatigue, muscle weakness, weight gain, hair loss and depression. The hair may be dry, and fingernails brittle and cracked. Many of these symptoms may be observed and attempts made to suppress or alleviate them without realizing that they indicate a thyroid problem. Until the thyroid problem is addressed, there will be no permanent improvement.

An acknowledged test for checking thyroid function, referred to as the Barnes Test is as follows. Keep a thermometer at bedside. Upon awakening, before any activity, check underarm temperature for five minutes. Do this for a number of mornings, recording the readings. A temperature consistently below 97.6° Fahrenheit and some of the above symptoms may indicate low thyroid function.

For this condition, reduce intake of foods which suppress the thyroid as mentioned above, while concentrating on seafood, kelp and other fruits such as apricots, dates and prunes and vegetables. High amounts of the B vitamins, iron, selenium and zinc, as well as vitamin C and E help the thyroid. Supplementing with thyroid glandular substance may also be beneficial. Avoid processed foods, white flour and sugar, fluoride, chlorine and any form of antihistamines.

## Toxic and Environmental Illness – TEI

*Thousands of chemicals and toxins are concocted and released into the environment.*

In recent decades, thousands of chemicals and toxic elements have been concocted and introduced into our environment. When I was a boy, the word environment generated thoughts of birds, trees and blue sky. Today that same word may invoke images of plastic containers, landfills and smog. A building used to be a place to go to escape from the elements. Today, buildings are often so full of toxic elements that we now have a problem referred to as "Sick Building Syndrome."

In my book, *Healthy Steps,* I describe a body detoxification program. Since that program was packaged, it has been used by tens of thousands. Many people who had total health frustration, including "incurable" diseases, have made dramatic recoveries.

A basic requirement for optimal health is a clean body, and often a sick body is an indication of a polluted body. Doesn't it make more sense to clean an engine choked by dirt than to try to keep fixing it? We must see that our bodies are a mirror image of the environment around us. If the food, water and air we take into our bodies is polluted, it is inevitable that our bodies will be polluted as well. Just like we must stop polluting and start cleaning up the environment around us, we must also stop polluting our bodies and start to clean up/detoxify them.

The fact that many chemicals are suspect in cancer development (these are referred to as carcinogenic) should motivate us all to detoxify. Besides, disease has little chance in a clean body, whereas it can thrive in a toxic body weakened by pollution. My most frequent response to hundreds of requests for health advise is "Start by cleansing your body. Health always works better in a clean body!"

*Health always works better in a clean body.*

It may also be necessary to consider the possibility of toxic reactions to chemicals in the workplace, or even in the home. Fumes from heating systems, electromagnetic radiation from power lines or appliances, as well as chemicals in carpets, paint, or furnishings may all be underlying contributors to health breakdown.

## Dietary Imbalance – DIM

"You are what you eat" is proving to be true even in the matter of disease and health breakdown. The converse, "you cannot be what you don't eat," may also be true. Nutritional deficiency can certainly undermine health. At the same time, we must be aware that a lack of variety and excessive amounts of certain types of foods, such as fats or refined carbohydrates, are also proven detriments to good health.

These matters have been thoroughly covered in Part Two, and the reader is advised to check there for more information on this subject. Many problems result from inadequate supply (deficiencies from a lack of proper food).

*One man's food can be another man's poison.*

It is also important to be aware that one man's food can be another man's poison. This again points toward the need for taking personal responsibility to know your body and to practice help yourself health care. Let me give an example. I just concluded a phone call where the conversation went somewhat as follows.

"Dr. Zehr, I'm trying to help a young man who has severe ulcerated colitis. He has diarrhea, is losing weight, and has no energy. Meanwhile, his immune system is so weak; he is always sickly. He was told that his bones are weak from lack of calcium. He has been put on various medications but none seem to help. Dr. Zehr, what could he take to help him?"

As usual, no thought or consideration had been given to his diet. I asked if he might be celiac, whereupon the caller replied, "What is that?"

I explained that a celiac has a severe allergy to the gluten found in wheat, oats, rye and barley. When gluten enters the intestine, the intestine reacts, becoming inflamed and shutting itself off to prevent absorption of the offending substance. The problem at this point is that protein and other vital nutrients cannot be absorbed either. The victim becomes malnourished and his bowels become inflamed.

The caller responded, "That sure sounds like his case, so what should he take?" Again we were caught in the "What do I take mode."

In my response I pointed out that aloe vera juice and green phytonutrients may generate healing. However, unless we address the matter of what is causing the irritation, little will be accomplished. It will be like hitting one's thumb each day, and trying to heal it each night.

The point is that a dietary imbalance may involve foods that are right or wrong for my body as well as foods that are simply good or bad. All of these factors need to be considered if we want to help ourselves to natural good health, rather then just alleviating and rearranging symptoms.

*First, get the body healthy, then let it deal with the problem.*

On the next few pages there is a list of over one hundred common diseases. In keeping with the principles outlined above, I suggest a probable disease category. Unless the disease is at a critical state, I would recommend addressing the underlying factors first. Over and over when I am asked, what to take for . . .(any of the following diseases), my answer is invariably the same: "Suppose, if instead of trying to attack that disease, we would help your body get healthy, then your body would be able to overcome the problem naturally. Only the body endowed with self-healing power by God can cure disease, if we give it a chance."

And how do we do this? We begin by being sure that we have Adequate Supply, Elimination, and Defense. Then, we identify the disease category and deal with those underlying conditions. By that time, recovery is well on its way. While there certainly are exceptions, and medical intervention may be necessary, this is surely the wisest place to begin. Medicine may bring faster symptomatic relief but leave permanent side effects, whereas the *help yourself* approach may be slower, but often results in full and permanent health recovery.

*See Chapter 7 for more on A SED.*

On the following pages is a list of over 100 common ailments with their corresponding disease categories.

> ### Key:
>
> The codes for disease categories are:
>
> **GN** – Genetic
>
> **AIR** – Allergy or Immune Related
>
> **YIR** – Yeast/Infection Related
>
> **TMR** – Thyroid/Metabolism Related
>
> **TEI** – Toxic/Environmental Illness
>
> **DIM** – Dietary Imbalance
>
> In all cases apply the A SED theory. For further details on each entry, see Chapter 19.

| *Name* | *Category* |
|--------|-----------|
| Acne | YIR, DIM |
| ADD | AIR, TEI, DIM |
| Age Spots | YIR, TEI |
| AIDS | YIR |
| Allergies | YIR, TEI, DIM |
| Alzheimer's | YIR, TMR, TEI |
| Arteriosclerosis | GN, DIM |
| Arthritis | AIR, DIM |
| Asthma | AIR, YIR |
| Autism | GN, TEI |
| | |
| Back pain | DIM |
| Bad breath | DIM |
| Bedsores | YIR, DIM |
| Bladder infection | YIR, DIM |
| Boils | YIR |
| Bronchitis | YIR, DIM |
| | |
| Cancer | TEI, AIR, DIM |
| Candidiasis | YIR, DIM |

| | |
|--------|-----------|
| Canker/cold sores | YIR |
| Carpal tunnel | TMR, YIR |
| Cataracts | YIR |
| Celiac | AIR, DIM |
| Cholesterol | DIM |
| Chronic fatigue | YIR, AIR, TMR |
| Cirrhosis | TEI, DIM |
| Colds | AIR, YIR |
| Colic | YIR |
| Colitis | AIR, YIR |
| Constipation | DIM |
| Crohn's disease | AIR, YIR |
| | |
| Dandruff | YIR, TEI |
| Depression | AIR, YIR, TEI, DIM |
| Dermatitis | YIR, AIR |
| Diabetes | GN, YIR, DIM |
| Diaper rash | YIR, DIM |
| Diarrhea | YIR, TEI, DIM |
| Diverticulitis | AIR, YIR, DIM |
| Dry eyes | AIR, YIR, TEI |
| | |
| Ear infection | YIR, AIR |
| Eczema | YIR, AIR, TEI |
| Edema | AIR |
| Emphysema | AIR, YIR |
| Endometriosis | YIR, AIR |
| Epilepsy | AIR, TEI |
| | |
| Fainting | TMR |
| Fatigue | YIR, AIR, TEI |
| Fibromyalgia | YIR, TEI |
| Flatulence | YIR, DIM |

| | |
|---|---|
| Flu | AIR, TEI, DIM |
| Food allergies | AIR |
| Fungal infection | YIR, DIM |
| | |
| Gallbladder disorders | DIM |
| Glaucoma | YIR |
| Gout | YIR, AIR, DIM |
| | |
| Hair loss | GN, YIR, DIM |
| Hay fever | AIR, YIR |
| Headaches | AIR, DIM |
| Heartburn | DIM, YIR |
| Heart disease | DIM, GN, TEI |
| Heel spurs | DIM |
| Hemorrhoids | DIM, AIR, YIR |
| Hepatitis | AIR |
| Hives | DIM, AIR, YIR |
| Hot flashes | TMR, YIR, AIR |
| Hyperactivity | DIM, YIR |
| Hypertension | GN, AIR, TMR |
| | |
| Impotence | YIR, TMR |
| Incontinence | YIR, AIR |
| Infection | AIR, YIR |
| Infertility | YIR, TEI, DIM |
| Insomnia | DIM, AIR, YIR |
| Irritable bowel syndrome | DIM, AIR |
| | |
| Kidney stones | DIM |
| | |
| Laryngitis | AIR, YIR |
| Leg cramps | DIM, YIR |
| Lupus | AIR, YIR |

| | |
|---|---|
| Lyme disease | AIR |
| | |
| Macular degeneration | YIR |
| Migraine | DIM, TEI, YIR |
| Mononucleosis | AIR, YIR |
| Morning sickness | DIM, YIR, TMR |
| Motion sickness | DIM |
| Multiple Sclerosis | YIR, AIR |
| Muscle cramps | DIM, YIR |
| | |
| Nail problems | DIM |
| Nausea | DIM, YIR, AIR |
| Nose bleeds | TMR, YIR |
| | |
| Obesity | DIM, TMR, TEI |
| Osteoporosis | DIM, TMR |
| | |
| Parasites | TMR, YIR |
| Parkinson's | AIR. YIR |
| Periodontal disease | DIM, YIR |
| PMS | TMR, YIR |
| Postpartum depression | YIR, AIR |
| Prostate problems | AIR, YIR |
| Psoriasis | YIR, AIR |
| | |
| Restless leg syndrome | TMR, AIR |
| Rheumatism | AIR, YIR, DIM |
| | |
| Shingles | YIR, TEI |
| Sinus infection | AIR, YIR |
| Sore throat | AIR, YIR |
| Sudden infant death syndrome | DIM, AIR |

Tonsillitis        AIR, YIR
Ulcers             DIM, YIR, AIR
Urinary problems YIR, AIR

Vaginitis          YIR
Varicose veins     DIM, YIR
Vitiligo           TMR, DIM

Warts              YIR, AIR

# Chapter 19

# Diseases and Natural Therapies

This chapter addresses the diseases listed in Chapter 18 and presents recommendations for natural therapies. The format used is as follows.

### Name

After the name or names of the problem, I describe very briefly how it is commonly identified.

*Background considerations:* Here, I list some possible reasons for the problem, such as deficiencies, toxins, allergens, etc.

*Possible disease category:* When appropriate, I indicate the disease category (as described in Chapter 18) which might need to be addressed for real restoration.

The codes are as follows:

GN -Genetic
AIR -Allergy or Immune Related
YIR -Yeast/Infection Related
TMR -Thyroid/Metabolism Related
TEI -Toxic/Environmental Illness
DIM - Dietary Imbalance

Take these background matters seriously. Dealing with them as described in Chapter 18 will often be a major step toward overcoming the particular problem.

*Home/folk remedies:* Here I list some folk or home remedies which seem to have some practical or historical validity.

*Natural therapies:* Nutritional supplements are listed here in order of importance, as well as herbal and other alternative therapies.

– Where specific amounts are not given, use amounts up to the high side of the helpful ranges shown in Chapter 11.

– Always remember the A SED theory as described in Chapter 7.

Some problems are dealt with in a less detailed format. In these cases, the reader will find the name in bold face, followed by the abbreviation for the possible disease category. There is also a brief description followed by some natural therapeutic suggestions.

For specific detoxification, immune support and yeast control programs see my book, *Healthy Steps.*

### Acne

Skin inflammation of the oil glands, appearing as blackheads, white heads, and pimples, on face, shoulders and elsewhere, mostly during puberty and adolescence.

*Background considerations:* When the rapidly growing and developing teenage body requires more nutrients than the typical junk food diet provides, the body may choose to use them to nourish maturing organs rather than to maintain healthy skin. This is true especially for minerals and essential fatty acids.

*Possible disease category:* YIR, DIM

*Home/folk remedies:* Bathe with warm milk, apply clay pack or aloe cream.

*Natural therapies*

*Diet:* Avoid sugar, white flour, caffeine, fried foods and dairy products.

*Nutrients:* vitamin A 50,000 IU, vitamin C 3000 mg., vitamin

E 440 IU, zinc 40 mg., flax seed oil, multiple minerals, B complex, and acidophilus.

*Herbs:* Alfalfa, echinacea, black currant seed oil, or evening primrose oil, chaparral, dandelion root, and yellow dock.

*Other:* Consider body detoxification and yeast control program.

## Attention Deficit Disorder – ADD          AIR, TEI, DIM

Increasing evidence is showing that these problems are often a result of reactions to chemicals or allergic reactions to food or environmental toxicity. ADD may also be related to dietary problems such as dairy allergies or mineral deficiencies.

Before accepting drugs, such as Ritalin with its plague of damaging side effects, be sure to be sure to consider

1) Checking for allergies to food or environmental toxins,

2) Detoxification as described earlier, and

3) Supplementation with minerals.

## Age Spots

Also called "liver spots," they appear as flat brown spots anywhere on the skin as the body ages. They are a result of waste buildup and free radical damage in skin cells.

*Background consideration:* Although age spots are considered harmless, they do indicate that the cells are accumulating waste matter which can damage not only the skin but also the brain and liver cells.

*Possible disease category:* YIR, TEI

*Natural therapies*

*Diet:* Green phytonutrients.

*Nutrients:* Antioxidants, especially vitamins C, E and A, selenium, CoQ10, pantothenic acid.

*Herbs:* Garlic, ginseng, gotu kola, licorice, sarsaparilla, dandelion root.

*Other:* Consider a liver cleanse and body detoxification.

## Acquired Immune Dysfunction – AIDS          YIR

The matter of AIDS is too complex to treat adequately in

this setting. At the risk of oversimplifying, I will share some points from our experience. While we have not had a total turnaround with confirmed cases, we have seen the ravages of this disease dramatically slowed down.

Overall, we must deal with the fact that the vitality of the immune system is being assaulted and only as we preserve and strengthen the immune system will we be successful in arresting this disease. Antioxidants are most important as are all immune strengthening nutrients and herbs.

In almost all cases of AIDS, yeast has also been devastating the body's resources. Dealing with this problem and eliminating any potential food allergies or any other immune stresses are important.

### Allergies                                   *YIR, TEI, DIM*
Be sure to see information on allergies page 109 and 196.

### Alzheimer's Disease
Also known as senile dementia. Alzheimer's is a progressive degenerative disease that attacks the brain, causing memory loss, and decreased mental and emotional function.

*Background considerations:* While Alzheimer's is an identifiable disease, it has become frequently misdiagnosed. Forgetfulness and memory loss may vary and be due to various influences. They should not be labeled too quickly as Alzheimer's. Forgetting where you put your shoes doesn't mean you have Alzheimer's, but forgetting that you wear shoes may. Research indicates that there may be multiple contributing factors. The most probable seem to be excessive levels of aluminium and mercury, and deficiencies of zinc, B12 and folic acid.

*Possible disease category:* YIR, TEI, TMR Also, check for possible cardiovascular problems.

*Natural therapies*

*Diet:* Phytonutrients, vegetable juices, high fiber.

*Nutrients:* CoQ10, lecithin, vitamins B6, C, E, selenium, zinc.

*Herbs:* Ginkgo biloba, gotu kola.

*Other:* Consider removing mercury amalgam dental fillings. Also consider detoxification and vascular cleansing either by EDTA (intravenous chelation) or oral chelation.

### Arteriosclerosis – see Heart Disease

### Arthritis

An inflammation of the joints, tendons, ligaments and cartilage. Arthritis means "fire in the joints." Effects range from slight pain and stiffness in the joints to crippling and excruciating pain to disability. In the past, arthritis was most common with the elderly. Now it affects all ages including many children. There are numerous forms of arthritis. The most common are osteoarthritis which results from the wear and tear and deterioration of the cartilage in each joint at the ends of the bones; and rheumatoid arthritis, an inflammation that attacks the synovial membranes of the joints. Other forms include gout, ankylosing spondylitis (AS), and systemic lupus erythematosus (SLE).

*Background considerations:* Sugar consumption, meat intake, especially pork, dairy, corn, wheat, citrus, and cereals all may aggravate arthritic tendencies

*Possible disease category:* AIR, DIM May relate to hormonal imbalance.

*Home/folk remedies:* Comfrey poultice, raw lemon rubs, copper bracelets, apple cider vinegar with honey, cod liver oil, hydrogen peroxide ($H_2O_2$) orally, cherries (especially for gout).

*Natural therapies*

*Diet:* Eliminate nightshade plants including peppers, potatoes, tomatoes, eggplant and tobacco for at least one month.

*Nutrients:* Cartilage, fish oil, flax seed oil, niacin, pantothenic acid, vitamin C, multiple minerals especially calcium and magnesium, trace minerals, glucosamine.

*Herbs:* Alfalfa, ginger, yucca, chaparral, devil's claw root, garlic, evening primrose oil.

*Other:* Try a vegetarian diet for one month. Drink vegetable juices and two quarts of distilled water daily. Acupuncture and accupressure may bring relief. Removal of mercury amalgam fillings has alleviated arthritis pain for some people. Some therapist believe that dealing with resentment and unresolved anger, or the need to control others may help some people deal with arthritic pain.

### Asthma

A chronic respiratory condition affecting breathing. Asthma is caused by an inflammation of the bronchials, the tubes that carry air within the lungs. Mostly affecting children, it involves wheezing, coughing, tightness of the chest and a feeling of suffocation. An asthma attack may be triggered by allergies, stress or an emotional state of fear or anxiety.

*Background considerations:* Since it is very much related to allergies, early breast-feeding instead of formula may reduce tendency. Other contributing factors may be exposure to cigarette smoke or other air pollutants, or milk allergy. There is some consideration that dehydration, inadequate water consumption, may aggravate this problem. Eating foods with sulfites (food preservatives) and artificial coloring products can also trigger asthma.

*Possible disease category:* AIR, YIR

*Home/folk remedies:* Drinking more water may relieve dehydration.

*Natural therapies*

*Diet:* Restrict salt intake, avoid food additives, check for dairy allergies.

*Nutrients:* Vitamins A, B6 400 mg., C 3000 mg., E 400 IU, magnesium.

*Herbs:* Mullein, hops, valerian root, chamomile, passion flower.

*Other:* Exercise

### Autism      *GN, TEI*

Children with autism do not react to their environment in a normal fashion. Their speech development is delayed or absent, often limited to babbling. They are generally unresponsive to affection and their behavior may range from silence to hyperactive aggression. Some become marginally self-sufficient, but most will need lifelong assistance.

Treating autism with megavitamin therapy has resulted in significantly improved speech, alertness, sleeping patterns and greater sociability. Most important are the B complex, especially vitamin B6, niacin, and pantothenic acid, vitamin C, and magnesium. Eliminating allergenic foods from the diet and avoiding chemical additives have also resulted in dramatic improvements.

There is reason to believe that there may be a connection between autism and infant vaccinations. See Chapter 15.

### Back Pain                                         DIM

Chiropractic and acupuncture treatments have generally proven to be most effective for dealing with back problems. Low deep back pain just above the hips may indicate kidney problems. Massage, accupressure and relaxation are all techniques that can be learned and used personally. Also, be sure that adequate minerals, especially magnesium, are taken.

### Bad Breath/ Halitosis                          YIR, DIM

Bad breath, also known as halitosis, may result from poor digestion, or infection of the mouth, teeth, nose or throat. It may also result from yeast infection or toxic chemicals in the body.

Begin by checking mouth hygiene and digestion. Chewing food more thoroughly, better food combining, and digestive enzyme supplements are ways digestion can be facilitated. After this, consider yeast control and body detoxification.

### Bedsores                                          YIR, DIM

For restoring damaged tissue, apply aloe vera gel. For faster healing, be sure patient gets at least 3,000 mg. vitamin C daily, administered in 500 mg. dosages throughout the day. Vitamin E 400 IU and zinc 80 mg. are also important.

### Bladder Infection / Bed-Wetting

Most common in women, bladder infections are caused by E. coli bacteria which usually begin in the vagina and migrate into the urinary tract. A strong burning sensation when urinating is the most common symptom.

*Background considerations:* Since bladder infection irritates primarily when one urinates, one may tend to reduce water intake. This is exactly the wrong thing to do. The more water one drinks and the more frequently one urinates, the less the bacteria will have opportunity to multiply and the sooner they will be flushed out. To avoid the possibility of transmitting bacteria from the bowel, wipe from front to back. Avoid aluminium cookware.

*Possible disease category:* YIR, DIM

*Home/folk remedies:* Cranberry juice, corn silk, honey, apple cider vinegar.

*Natural therapies*

*Diet:* Avoid citrus fruits, caffeine, carbonated beverages and alcohol.

*Nutrients:* Vitamin C 3000 mg., calcium, magnesium, zinc.

*Herbs:* Uva ursi, garlic, parsley.

*Other:* Acidophilus.

### Boils                                                                                   YIR, TEI

A boil is an infected nodule of the skin where swelling and redness may be followed by a central core eruption of pus. A boil is the body's attempt to rid itself of impurities. Activate detoxification, yeast control and better nutrition; especially zinc and vitamins A, C and E are important. More water will also help the body to stay clean internally.

Take vitamin C 3000 mg. daily, apply vitamin A topically and apply hot compresses to relieve pain and promote healing.

### Bronchitis                                                                             YIR, DIM

Be sure that possible yeast infection is under control. In the meantime, take at least 4000 mg. vitamin C, 20000 IU Beta

Carotene and drink 2 to 3 quarts of pure water daily. Eucalyptus, echinacea, fenugreek or ginger herbs may be helpful. An old home remedy was to apply a compress of chopped onions mixed with lard to the chest at night. Another home remedy is to make a compress of hot mustard.

## Cancer

A condition where cells in the body stop functioning, maturing and replacing themselves in a normal orderly way. The cells begin to multiply uncontrollably and form a tumor mass which then siphons energy and nourishment from the body for its own supply. If left unchecked, these abnormal cells may cause more tumors throughout the body as they circulate.

*Background considerations:* Every cell in the human body has a limited life span. As this time ends, the cell must be replaced identically in content and number. If the cell is replaced in an erratic way or millions of times, mutant cells result. When the body is loaded with toxicity, the immune system gets frustrated and can no longer maintain its control over these mutant cells. Clumping together to form a tumor, they may become destructive and eventually fatal.

Selenium deficiency has been conclusively demonstrated to be a significant factor in susceptibility to cancer. Conversely, selenium supplementation has been shown to be effective for cancer prevention and also for cancer recovery.

By addressing the following three areas, we have seen numerous victims overcome cancer.

1) The growth of the tumor must be arrested.
2) The toxicity level in the body must be lowered.
3) The immune system must be supplied and activated.

*Possible disease category:* TEI, AIR, DIM Since toxic load may lie behind cancer, a total body cleanse as explained elsewhere is often a crucial factor.

*Home/folk remedies:* Shark or bovine cartilage can arrest cancer's growth, since it seems to restrict the growth of new tissue. Essiac is a herbal remedy given to René Caisse by natives. It is a blood purifier and seems to promote antitumor and cleansing activity. Since the formula has been disclosed, it is now available under various labels. Be sure that it contains the four basic ingredients: burdock root, sheep sorrel, turkey rhubarb root and slippery elm bark. Aloe vera juice can help to activate the immune system to overcome cancer.

*Natural therapies*

*Diet:* Fresh carrot/vegetable juice, greens, no animal products.

*Nutrients:* Vitamin C 5000 mg., selenium 200 mcg., beta carotene.

*Herbs:* Aloe vera, pau d'arco, garlic, chaparral.

*Other:* Avoid all chemicals, macrobiotic diet may be helpful.

## Candidiasis

This condition results from Candida Albicans, a type of yeast-like fungus which inhabits the intestine (especially the colon), the genital tract, respiratory tract, mouth, nose, ears, and throat. While this fungus normally lives in balance with other bacteria and yeast in the body, it is very aggressive and will invade any unguarded territory. When it does, it severely frustrates the immune system and sets the stage for many symptoms.

The use of antibiotics, X-rays, poor diet and high sugar consumption create ideal conditions for Candida Albicans to thrive.

*Possible disease category:* YIR, DIM. This is the underlying monster referred to under the category YIR. Its symptoms are numerous and include: constipation, diarrhea, colitis, canker sores, joint pain, sore throat, vaginitis, acne, arthritis, depression, hyperactivity and more.

*Home/folk remedies:* Acidophilus, garlic, body detoxification.

*Natural therapies*

*Diet:* Sugar and alcohol must be avoided

*Nutrients:* Caprylic acid, vitamin C, multivitamin minerals

*Herbs:* Pau d'arco, grapefruit seed extract.

*Other:* For a full discussion of the yeast problem and a comprehensive program, see *Healthy Steps,* chapter 6.

### Canker / Cold Sores                                    YIR

Avoid sugar. Take lysine 1500 mg, acidophilus, B complex, vitamin E, niacin, zinc.

### Carpal Tunnel Syndrome                          TMR, YIR

The compression of the nerve in the wrist produces numbness, tingling, pain and weakness of the fingers. Sometimes the condition can be relieved naturally but sometimes surgical correction may be required.

Vitamin B6 deficiency may be involved, as may low thyroid, ingestion of chemical food additives, dyes and preservatives. Yeast infection may aggravate the problem. Mineral supplements are also helpful.

### Cataracts                                              YIR

Cataracts, an opaqueness or cloud that forms over the lens of the eye, is a leading cause of blindness. It may be related to degenerative changes that occur with aging. It may also be due, especially in diabetics, to consumption of milk products. Drugs, stress, pollution and poor diet may also produce the disease.

Eating a diet rich in leafy green vegetables and supplementing with vitamins A, C, D, E, B complex and minerals are helpful. The herb eyebright has been used for generations and good results are still being experienced.

### Celiac Disease

Celiac disease is an often overlooked ailment caused by a severe intolerance to gluten. Gluten is found in wheat, oats, barley, and rye. When gluten irritates the sensitive lining of the intestine it becomes inflamed and unable to absorb vital nutritional elements, especially protein. Severe malnutrition and diarrhea may result even though the patient is eating well.

*Background considerations:* Celiac symptoms may include diarrhea, foul smelling stools, nausea, abdominal swelling, weight loss, skin irritation, and may often be misdiagnosed as irritable bowel syndrome or colitis. It may be found in children or adults and may make the victim more susceptible to schizophrenia.

*Possible disease category:* AIR, DIM It may also be yeast related.

*Home/folk remedies:* Relatively new disorder. None commonly used.

*Natural therapies:* Observe strict dietary guidelines.

*Diet:* Eat absolutely no gluten-containing grains: wheat, oats, barley or rye. No sugar, processed foods or dairy products.

*Nutrients:* B vitamins, vitamin K, multivitamin minerals, protein such as in soya or spirulina.

*Herbs:* Spirulina, alfalfa, kelp.

*Other:* Sunflower seeds, nuts.

### Cholesterol                                          DIM

Probably the most controversial and most confusing topic in health is cholesterol. To bring some light to this matter, let's begin with some facts. First, let's be aware that the body produces all the cholesterol it needs. And, whether you get it in your diet or not, the body still produces the amount necessary. Therefore, whatever you get in your food is extra; nutritionally it is unnecessary, and potentially harmful.

The body, however, does need cholesterol. It is important for manufacturing steroids or cortisone-like hormones; it helps the liver produce bile; and it is a building block for body tissues. The problem arises when there is too much cholesterol, for then it is deposited inside the walls of the arteries creating a lack of oxygen to the heart muscle.

Since blood is water based and cholesterol is a fatty substance, it can not be mixed with blood so it must be packaged into molecules called lipoproteins. These lipoproteins move the cholesterol throughout the body to where it is needed and remove it from where it is not needed.

Generally speaking, LDL (low density lipoprotein) often referred to as the bad cholesterol, delivers the cholesterol, whereas, HDL (high density lipoprotein) known as the good cholesterol helps to remove and transport cholesterol to the liver for excretion. This may be an oversimplification of the problem, but it gets to the basic idea.

High cholesterol, 210 or above, significantly increases the possibility of heart disease, and high amounts of cholesterol in the colon increase the risk of cancer there. Food cholesterol that has been heated or exposed to oxygen is altered by dangerous free radicals.

So, what can we do? Remember that only animal products (meat, especially organ meats and eggs which often appear in baked goods) contain cholesterol. Limit or cut these out and most of the problem will be gone. Further, be aware that vitamin C greatly reduces the potential damage of cholesterol in the arteries. Take at least 2000 mg. daily for adequate protection. Get adequate fiber to remove cholesterol from the intestines and colon quickly. And finally, stop looking for a magic, "what to take" bullet. If you eat right, have a clean and healthy body and reduce stress, then forget about the numbers and enjoy a peaceful, long, healthy life.

## Chronic Fatigue Syndrome

Chronic Fatigue Syndrome (CFS) earlier known as Epstein Bar Virus (EBV) has become an increasingly common ailment in recent years. The victim is chronically tired, sleeps for hours but does not feel rested. Sore throat, depression, mood swings, loss of appetite, difficulty concentrating, headaches and aching joints are just some of the symptoms. The primary symptom, however, is constant fatigue.

*Background considerations:* The problem is much more common in women. Antibiotics are of little value and only a strong immune system can bring this condition under control. Chronic mercury poisoning from dental fillings may be involved and removal is sometimes advised.

*Possible disease category:* YIR, AIR, TMR It may be yeast related and aggravated by toxicity. A detoxification and yeast control program may be major steps in recovery.

*Home/folk remedies:* None. Relatively new disorder.

*Natural therapies:* Fresh greens and mild exercise out-of-doors.

*Diet:* Avoid sugar, dairy, processed foods. Eat fresh raw vegetables and fruits, acidophilus and yogurt.

*Nutrients:* Beta Carotene, vitamins C, and B complex, selenium, pantothenic acid, CoQ10.

*Herbs:* Garlic, spirulina, echinacea, burdock root.

*Other:* Drink at least eight glasses of water daily, do a detoxification program.

### Cirrhosis of the Liver        TEI, DIM

Cirrhosis of the liver is a condition where the cells of the liver have hardened and the liver is unable to maintain its function of blood cleansing. This condition is often due to alcoholism, viral hepatitis or severe malnutrition.

Body detoxification, fresh vegetable juices, non-animal protein and the elimination of alcohol, sugar, dairy and animal products will help the body enact a slow recovery.

### Colds        AIR, YIR

The common cold, a viral infection of the upper respiratory tract, is usually expressed by congestion, coughing, headache, fever, sneezing and watery eyes. Because there are numerous cold viruses, it is impossible to find a specific medication. Stress, fatigue, yeast infection, poor diet and a toxic body all weaken the body's resistance and make one more susceptible to "catching" a cold.

The best protection is a strong immune system, and that is why some of us rarely have a cold. I may have one about every third year or less.

If "hit" with a cold, take high doses of vitamin A (4000 IU) and vitamin C 500 mg. every two hours. Also, increase zinc intake. If we do this when we first sense a cold coming, we can greatly reduce the severity. If we wait until the cold has fully hit us, then recovery will be much slower.

Keeping the immune system strong, our bodies clean, taking a good supplement program and eating right are the best ways to deal with colds, before they deal with us.

## Colic                                    YIR, DIM

Colic refers to conditions of gas or other digestive discomfort in infants. Breast milk is much better tolerated, but a colicky baby may be reacting to something the mother has eaten.

According to Dr. Lendon Smith, up to 50 percent of infants are allergic to cow's milk which may result in colic, diarrhea, rashes, ear infections and asthma. He has found that a mixture of apple cider and water, mixed one teaspoon per 8 ounces can be a helpful remedy. A mild mix of dill seed and water can also be helpful.

## Colitis – see Diverticulitis and Crohn's Disease

## Constipation                              DIM

Constipation is characterized by slow and inadequate movement of waste material from the colon and bowel. It may result in hemorrhoids, gas, insomnia, varicose veins, diverticulitis, and bowel cancer. The primary reasons for this disorder are insufficient water, inadequate fiber, and lack of exercise.

Drinking more water, and taking bran or psyllium husks, flaxseed, aloe vera juice, green juice, alfalfa, cascara sagrada or acidophilus are natural ways to correct this problem.

## Crohn's Disease

Crohn's disease, a chronic inflammation of the digestive tract; it seems to strike around age twenty.

*Background considerations:* The risk is increased with a history of food allergies and may be aggravated by the same. Symptoms include diarrhea, cramping, lower abdominal pain, fever, poor absorption, possible anemia, and loss of energy and weight. Lack of nutrient absorption may weaken the immune system and could cause iron deficiency anemia.

*Possible disease category:* AIR, YIR

*Home/folk remedies:* Aloe vera

*Natural therapies*
*Diet:* Aloe vera, fresh vegetables, no meat or dairy.
*Nutrients:* Acidophilus, vitamins B complex, C, E.
*Herbs:* Garlic, spirulina, green phytonutrients.
*Other:* Avoid spicy, fried or greasy foods, caffeine, alcohol, dairy products, carbonated drinks, chocolate and animal products.

### Dandruff                                                    YIR, TEI

Those embarrassing "snow flakes" which show up on your shoulders seem to be more noticeable than your new black suit. While they simply may be dry skin flakes from the scalp, treated shampoos and more or less frequent washing usually does not help significantly.

More results are usually realized from adjusting diet. Avoid fried foods, dairy products, sugar, white flour, chocolate, nuts and seafood. Eat fresh and raw fruits and vegetables. For herbal help, try dandelion, goldenseal, and use chaparral as a hair rinse. Also include extra vitamins A, B complex, C and selenium.

### Depression                                    AIR, YIR, TEI, DIM

Sadness comes to us all on occasion, but depression involves frequent and long lasting feelings of sadness and despair. It may include insomnia, lack of appetite, disinterest in otherwise enjoyable activities, irritability, moodiness, loss of self esteem and feelings of hopelessness and guilt.

Depression may be the result of an imbalance of brain chemicals. This could be instigated by toxins in the body, or allergic reactions to chemicals or even food. It may be greatly aggravated by yeast overgrowth. All of these areas and a healthy diet should be tried before medications are used.

The most helpful vitamins and herbs are: vitamin B complex, lecithin, choline, inositol, all minerals, vitamin C, chamomile, evening primrose oil, and feverfew.

## Dermatitis

Chronic itching/inflammation of the skin, may include patches of redness, weeping fluid and scaling with blisters.

*Background considerations:* May be aggravated by yeast problem, address this first.

*Possible disease category:* YIR, AIR

*Home/folk remedies:* Sauerkraut, yogurt, baking soda bath – one cup per tub full.

*Natural therapies*

*Diet:* Identify and avoid food allergies especially milk, eggs and wheat. Consider a gluten free diet. See celiac disease.

*Nutrients:* Vitamin E, vitamin C, essential fatty acids, zinc, acidophilus, B complex, biotin, multi-minerals.

*Herbs:* Flax seed, evening primrose oil.

*Other:* Consider possibility of body or laundry soap allergy. Apply aloe vera or evening primrose oil topically.

## Diabetes

A disorder in which the body is not properly able to process sugar and make it available to be "burned" in the cells as fuel for life, energy and health maintenance. There are two different forms.

Type I, formerly called juvenile diabetes, results from a lack of insulin, the hormone that allows cells to take up glucose (sugar) circulating in the bloodstream.

Also known as insulin dependent diabetes mellitus, it is caused by damage to the pancreas which then cannot adequately produce the necessary insulin.

Type II, or non-insulin-dependent diabetes mellitus also known as adult onset diabetes, occurs when sugar cannot get inside the cells. This is referred to as insulin resistance, because the receptor sites on the membranes of the cells don't allow sugar inside.

In both types there is too much sugar in the blood and this puts tremendous stress on the body, so that other disease potential such as poor wound healing, heart disease, vision loss and poor circulation is increased.

*Background considerations:* While the exact cause of diabetes is not fully understood, it occurs much more in "western diet" countries and can be significantly helped by dietary changes as well as with supplementation. Some studies indicate that lack of breast-feeding, or too early introduction of cows milk or solid foods, (before four months) may increase the possibility of diabetes.

*Possible disease category:* GN, YIR, DIM May be related to obesity.

*Home/folk remedies:* Blueberry leaf tea, alfalfa tea, comfrey, dandelion, guar gum, pectin, ginseng.

*Natural therapies:* Eat high fiber, low protein, exercise.

*Diet:* The most significant help possible comes through dietary adjustments.

– Avoid refined carbohydrates, all forms of sugars or honey.

– Eat complex carbohydrate, high fiber, fresh fruits and vegetables, green beans, cucumber, garlic, mushrooms, beets, whole grains, oatmeal, brown rice, cornmeal, beans, spinach, green leafy vegetables, celery, kelp.

– Keep fats to a minimum – small amounts of fish and chicken.

– Eat smaller meals frequently, rather than large meals.

– Drink lots of water, but not with meals.

*Nutrients:* Vitamin C 2000 mg, vitamin E 400 IU, magnesium 500 mg, calcium 1000 mg, chromium 200 mcg, B complex 100 mg, CoQ10 60 mg, multi-mineral.

*Herbs:* Garlic, onions, blueberry leaves, fenugreek, hawthorn berry, ginkgo Biloba.

*Other:* Get adequate rest and exercise, eat no junk food.

### Diaper Rash                                                    YIR, DIM

The way to avoid diaper rash is to eliminate the diaper. Just kidding! Certainly, a clean dry diaper is important. A diaper with urine and stool produces ammonia and makes diaper rash worse. If possible avoid plastic liners, as they trap moisture. A deficiency of zinc may be involved, 10 mg of crushed zinc in babies food may help.

Breast-fed babies have less diaper rash. Cool blow drying

the baby's bottom may help. Cornstarch is helpful but do not use baking soda or vaseline as it doesn't allow the skin to breathe. Check for possible dairy allergy. Diaper rash may also be a yeast problem aggravated by sugar intake.

### Diarrhea                                    YIR, TEI, DIM

The loose, watery, frequent bowel movements called diarrhea are the body's way of trying to quickly expel irritating toxicity from the bowel. It may be caused by virus, bacteria, chemicals, incomplete digestion, toxic food, parasites or allergens. So, it is not simply a matter of trying to stop it. Since diarrhea can quickly dehydrate the body, drinking clean water is advised.

Attempt to determine and alleviate the underlying problem. Be sure there is adequate fiber in the diet. Carob, acidophilus or "green" drinks may bring improvement. Digestive enzymes, vitamins B, C, D and E, charcoal tablets, kelp, slippery elm, chamomile and raspberry leaves may also help. Do not consume milk products.

Brown rice cooked with extra water and mixed with banana is gentle on the system and may help to re-establish normal bowel function.

### Diverticulitis                              AIR, YIR, DIM

Diverticula are small pouch-like growths that develop in the walls of the colon. High fat and red meat consumption weakens the colon walls. If there is a lack of fiber or constipation, the pressure produces these sacs. If they become infected, pain, cramping and tenderness on the left side of the abdomen probably indicate diverticulitis.

Avoid red meat; consume high fiber, especially oat bran and high fiber fruit, like blackberries, raspberries and blueberries. Beans and peas are good sources of fiber. Acidophilus, aloe vera, garlic and essential fatty acids are helpful.

### Dry Eyes                                    AIR, YIR, TEI

Water in our eyes is not only necessary for crying, but also for constant lubrication and natural cleansing. When our eyes do not produce adequate water, they become dry, can irritating, and may even pose a serious health problem. Possible reasons for this condition are medications, especially diuretics, antihistamines or antidepressants, vitamin A deficiency and lack of humidity.

Check for allergies; supplement with vitamin A; get a humidifier; drink lots of juice and water while traveling on planes; blink your eyes frequently and consider using eye drops. The herb eyebright has been historically used and often proven helpful for eye conditions, even for cataracts.

### Ear Infection

Infection of the middle ear is quite common among children. It usually results from the spread of bacteria from an infection in the nose or throat although food allergies may also play a part. Symptoms include ear pain, fullness in the ear, hearing loss, discharge from the ear and fever.

*Background considerations:* Often associated with early formula feeding. Breast-feeding may be one of the best protections against ear infection. Cows milk can be an irritation to the eustachian tubes and a common allergen. Unsanitary conditions or low immunity are often contributing factors.

*Possible disease category:* YIR, AIR

*Home/folk remedies:* Use garlic oil as an ear drop. Clay pack used externally.

*Natural therapies:* Chew garlic cloves. Use mild hydrogen peroxide as ear drops.

*Diet:* Avoid sugar and cows milk, and all other foods the child may be allergic to. The most common are dairy product, eggs, wheat, corn, oranges and peanut butter.

*Nutrients:* Vitamins A, E, C and B complex, zinc, manganese.

*Herbs*: Echinacea, garlic, evening primrose oil, OPC.

*Other:* Prolonged breast-feeding, at least six months, offers the child's immune system a chance to build up, and becomes an invaluable protection against all disease both in childhood and thereafter.

### Eczema

A chronic skin irritation often expressing itself with itching, rash and sometimes open weeping.

*Background considerations:* May be activated by chlorinated water, nickel from earring posts (use only stainless steel), antiperspirants, hair dyes and sprays or acrylic manicure products. Laundry or bath soap and synthetic fibers in clothing or bedding may be aggravating factors. Orange juice, eggs, peanuts, wheat and milk also have been implicated as eczema aggravators in children. All of this calls for careful detective work. While topical applications may soothe the irritation, they rarely address the real problem.

*Possible disease category:* YIR, AIR, TEI

*Home/folk remedies:* Bathe in finely ground colloidal oatmeal. Apply Aloe Vera.

*Natural therapies*

*Diet:* Avoid fried foods, animal fats and processed meats and all preservatives. Concentrate on fresh fruit and vegetables.

*Nutrients:* Vitamins A, E and B complex with extra B12, zinc.

*Herbs:* Primrose oil, comfrey, kelp, flax seed, aloe vera topical and internal, chaparral, and red clover.

*Other:* Avoid excess sunshine. Drink plenty of pure water and fresh juices.

### Edema                                        AIR

Sometimes called dropsy, edema is a fluid accumulation, especially in the feet and ankles. It probably involves kidney, bladder or liver problems. Check for allergies and be sure that yeast is under control. It may indicate a protein deficiency, try spirulina as an excellent non-animal source of protein. Herbs, alfalfa, horsetail, corn silk, or dandelion may be helpful. Eat fresh raw foods and avoid salt, dairy, fried foods, sugar, caffeine, alcohol, and pickled foods.

### Emphysema                                    AIR, YIR

A severe respiratory ailment where the lungs have lost elasticity and breathing becomes difficult especially upon exertion. Most cases are a result of smoking and can be recovered from only if smoking is avoided. Body detoxification, improved diet and following asthma suggestions can provide significant improvement.

### Endometriosis

Endometriosis is a condition that results from the presence of actively growing and functioning endometrial tissue in areas outside the uterus. The tissue can be widespread including the ovaries, urinary bladder and beyond. The most common symptom is painful menstrual periods, although many women report no discomfort.

*Background considerations:* Low immune function, yeast overgrowth and nutritional imbalance may increase susceptibility.

*Possible disease category:* YIR, AIR Control of yeast and building up immunity are crucial for natural recovery.

*Home/folk remedies:* Green vegetables, spirulina, barley green.

*Natural therapies*

*Diet:* Avoid caffeine, sugar, animal products and fast food. Eat raw fruits, vegetables, nuts, whole grains.

*Nutrients:* Iodine, omega-3, vitamin E, C, minerals.

*Herbs:* Dong quai, raspberry leaves, ginseng.

*Other:* Drink eight glasses of water daily.

### Epilepsy

Epilepsy is expressed by seizures caused by electrical disturbances in the nerve cells of the brain. Petit mal seizures are mild and may be evidenced only by a blank staring into space while twitching slightly. Grand mal seizures are more extreme. The person afflicted may fall to the ground, become unconscious and have convulsions for two to five minutes. This is followed by confusion, fatigue or memory loss.

*Background considerations:* Epilepsy can be caused by infection, meningitis, rickets, rabies, tetanus, malnutrition, hypoglycemia, head injuries, high fever, allergies, or scar tissue.

Studies have associated aspartame with seizures. Lead

poisoning and aluminium toxicity, and nitrites found in processed meats such as hot dogs may also contribute to the problem. Years ago, children eating baby food deficient in vitamin B6 developed severe convulsions.

*Possible disease category:* AIR, TEI

*Home/folk remedies:* Eat soured milk products.

*Natural therapies*

*Diet:* Fresh fruits and vegetables, including juices, olive oil. Avoid alcohol, animal products, caffeine, aspartame, refined sugar and nicotine.

*Nutrients:* B complex, B6, magnesium, manganese, chromium.

*Herbs:* Valerian, mistletoe, kelp.

*Other:* Stay away from pesticides and all chemicals. Exercise and avoid stress.

## Fainting                                              TMR

Consider the possibility of low blood sugar, low blood pressure, allergies, anemia, or thyroid disorder. Eat a whole foods diet with adequate protein such as spirulina and soya products supplemented with magnesium, iron, B complex, pantothenic acid and vitamin C.

If you feel faint, place head low or between knees, get plenty of fresh air, hold peppermint or black pepper under nose.

## Fatigue– see Chronic Fatigue Syndrome   YIR, AIR, TEI

## Fibromyalgia

A relatively new term given to a variety of painful symptoms; often misdiagnosed as MS, gout, arthritis, chronic fatigue, or acute anxiety. An accurate test has not been agreed upon, but fibromyalgia is assumed if pain is felt in at least 10 of 18 "tender points" when pressure is applied. Fatigue, morning stiffness, headaches, depression, tingling of arms and legs, and pain all over may all be involved in this condition.

The pain may be present in any fibromuscular tissue, most common in the lower portion of the back of the skull, neck, shoulders, chest, low back and thighs. For some the pain is so constant and debilitating that normal activities are no longer possible. Some believe that fibromyalgia is a modern form of what was earlier called rheumatism.

*Background considerations:* Studies indicate that people who are under physical and mental stress, anxious, tense and striving, and those who are perfectionists are more likely to develop fibromyalgia. Adrenal exhaustion is almost always involved.

*Possible disease category:* YIR, TEI Stress, yeast overgrowth and allergies all contribute to a situation where fibromyalgia may develop.

*Home/folk remedies:* Massage, exercise.

*Natural therapies*

*Diet:* Fresh fruits, vegetables, avoid, caffeine, meat, dairy, alcohol, processed foods.

*Nutrients:* Beta Carotene, vitamin B12, vitamin E, pantothenic acid, folic acid, selenium, zinc, grape seed extract, and CoQ10.

*Herbs:* Echinacea, ginger, peppermint tea, aloe vera.

*Other:* See program for Chronic Fatigue in Chapter 7 of *Healthy Steps*.

### Flatulence                                            YIR, DIM

Although some foods like beans may have a greater tendency toward producing gas, flatulence is primarily a result of poor digestion, food intolerance and/or poor food combining.

When vegetables and protein are consumed, they require a number of hours for proper digestion. If this is followed immediately by fruit or refined carbohydrates, digestion is frustrated and gas may well result. Eat foods from the various groups separately as explained under food combining in Chapter 9.

For beans, broccoli, and cabbage, a digestive enzyme such as "Beano" may be helpful. Charcoal, herbs like ginger, clove, allspice, and oils from anise seed, caraway, fennel or peppermint are good natural remedies. Also check for common food allergies.

## Flu                                    AIR, TEI, DIM

"Catching" the flu is a result of being exposed to a flu virus and not having the immediate immune response to resist it. Once one has the flu, it pretty much must run its course. The secret for avoiding the flu does not come by running from it, nor by a flu vaccination, but by a good diet and a strong immune system.

Getting extra sleep, cutting out sugar consumption, drinking large amounts of water, juices and broth, and 1000-2,000 mg vitamin C intake will help the body to overcome by strengthening the immune system and enhancing detoxification.

## Food Allergies – see Chapters 9and 17.

## Fungal Infection – see Candidiasis and Warts YIR, DIM

## Gallbladder Disorders                        DIM

This small organ located under the liver acts as a reservoir to store bile which the body uses to digest fats. Sometimes the cholesterol contained in the bile crystallizes to form gallstones. Some patients with gallstones have no symptoms, but when a stone blocks the bile duct, severe pain, nausea, and vomiting may occur.

Eat fresh foods, avoid animal fats and surgery if possible. A home remedy that has proven helpful to many is as follows: For two days do not eat; then drink only water and pure whole apple juice for two days. On the morning of the third day, take two ounces of extra virgin olive oil. Lie on your left side and rest. Within a short time you will pass soft green pebbles of bile and softened stones.

## Glaucoma – see Macular Degeneration          YIR

## Gout                                     YIR, DIM

When too much uric acid occurs in the body it begins to crystallize and gout results. Experienced mostly by males, it may show up in the joints, fingers, large toe or elsewhere. It is related to poor protein metabolism, obesity, and purine rich foods such as alcohol, caffeine, meat, mushrooms, and asparagus. Pastries and sugar products should also be avoided. Fruits, vegetables and clean drinking water as well as vitamin and mineral supplements are important. Take spirulina as a non-animal protein source.

A long famous home remedy is to eat a bowl full of cherries or strawberries since they neutralize uric acid.

### Hair Loss                                           GN, TEI, YIR

Hair loss or baldness is referred to as alopecia. While baldness in men may be partially determined by heredity, other factors are also involved. These include poor circulation, poor diet, radiation, skin disease, iron deficiency, drugs, stress, and high levels of toxicity. Rectifying any of these conditions is helpful.

Important supplements are biotin, B complex, essential fatty acids, vitamin C, E, CoQ10, and PABA for gray hair recovery. Massage the scalp daily. Rinsing hair with apple cider vinegar or aloe vera juice may be helpful. Tight braids, hair dyes, hot rollers, and harsh chemical dyes may all contribute to hair loss. Be aware that women often have some loss of hair after pregnancy. It is normal to lose up to 100 hairs per day. If you lose more than 100 hairs beware!

### Hay Fever                                           AIR, YIR, TEI

Hay fever, also known as allergic rhinitis, affects up to ten percent of the population. It is commonly associated with pollen although it may also be related to dust, dog and cat dander, mold spore, insect bites or perfume. Hay fever is a disorder of the immune system and should primarily be addressed by detoxification and immune support.

Check for allergies, yeast, and environmental toxins. Avoid perfumes, scented soaps, house dust, mold, and chemicals. CoQ10, vitamins A, B, C and E, fresh fruits and vegetables can help support the immune system. See also Asthma.

## Headache                                    DIM, TEI, YIR

Headaches may be a response to stress, a reaction to wheat, dairy, sugar, chocolate, MSG or any number of preservatives, etc. A low headache at the back of the head may be triggered by constipation. Begin by clearing up the diet, checking allergies as indicated earlier, and dealing with constipation and yeast.

Most headaches can be relieved within minutes by applying finger pressure to the "tender points" on the shoulders, neck, temples, and forehead. Niacin along with herbs, including feverfew, peppermint, goldenseal, and lobelia, may be helpful. All of the above also applies to migraines.

## Heartburn                                        DIM, YIR

The condition referred to as heartburn is primarily a burning sensation in the upper stomach and lower esophagus. This occurs when hydrochloric acid, a powerful stomach acid backs, up into the esophagus. It is caused by poor digestion, and may be the result of eating too many spicy, fatty or fried foods, consuming too much alcohol, coffee, chocolate, and tomato, or as a result of food allergies.

Chew your food well. Check food combining. Take aloe vera juice, proteolytic enzymes, or apple cider vinegar. If you take a tablespoon full of apple cider vinegar or lemon juice and the heartburn goes away, then you need more hydrochloric acid. If it makes the symptoms more intense, then you have too much acid.

## Heart Disease                               DIM, GN, TEI

The heart is an amazing organ which acts as a pump. It pumps about 1000 gallons of blood through 60,000 miles of blood vessels by pumping 100,000 times each day. It is the most crucial organ of the human body. Heart disease has become the number one killer in America. Many people who died from this disease did not even know they had it.

The main problem lies in the arteries, those vessels which bring blood loaded with fresh oxygen to supply the heart muscles. When these arteries get congested and partially blocked, it is no longer possible for adequate oxygen to be brought to the heart and a heart attack, often referred to as angina, occurs. This may express itself with severe chest pain. The heart may be damaged or the consequences may be almost immediate death.

*Background considerations:* Even though a heart attack may be sudden, the conditions develop over a period of time. When there is too much fat in the blood, the red blood cells clump together. The walls are damaged allowing fat, cholesterol, and calcium to enter into the muscular wall of the artery. As this problem progresses, the arteries become more blocked, aggravated by free radicals and poor diet. When exertion demands more output from the heart, sufficient oxygenated blood is not available and an attack ensues.

*Possible disease category:* DIM, GN, TEI There is no doubt that diet plays a major role in the development of this problem and it must be central in a recovery plan. Free radicals resulting from rancid fats and chemicals are crucial in heart disease and must be dealt with by making dietary adjustments and taking antioxidants.

*Home/folk remedies:* Garlic by the clove, red beet juice, kelp, apple cider vinegar.

*Natural therapies:* Complete body detoxification.

*Diet:* Avoid all animal fats, dairy products, eat fresh fruits and vegetables.

*Nutrients:* Vitamins E and C, selenium, all antioxidants, magnesium, CoQ10.

*Herbs:* Cayenne, garlic, kelp, dandelion, hawthorn berries, and ginkgo biloba.

*Other:* Former heart surgeon, Dr. Julian Whitaker, insists that heart surgery is much less effective and far more dangerous than nutritional intervention. The supplement program outlined in *Healthy Steps* has helped many to recovery from circulatory problems.

### Heel Spurs                                        DIM

A heel or bone spur is a hard pointed growth on the bone of the heel or elsewhere. It is made up of calcium deposits and is often related to arthritis, neuritis, or alkalosis. Strange as it may sound, taking minerals especially a natural source calcium may help the spur to dissolve.

Drink distilled water, no citrus, coffee, sugar, or alcohol. Take mineral supplements and digestive enzymes to enhance proper absorption.

### Hemorrhoids                               DIM, AIR, YIR

Swollen veins around the anus that may protrude out of the rectum or remain inside can cause great pain and discomfort. They are often related to inadequate fiber, constipation, lack of exercise, heavy lifting, prolonged periods of sitting or allergies. Check allergies, increase fiber intake and exercise. Flax seed, white oak bark, and vitamin E are helpful. Using raw potato or garlic cloves as a suppository and taking a sitz bath in hot epsom salt water are among the folk remedies used.

### Hot Flashes                               TMR, YIR, AIR

Hot flashes are defined as recurrent, transient periods of flushing, sweating sensations of heat, often including heart palpitations. This is a result of hormonal changes during the time when a woman's body stops ovulating. It usually occurs between age 45 and 52.

While estrogen production may drop, the hormone does not disappear. The body has ways to compensate with other hormones for the reduction in estrogen supply. The body should be able to adjust if the diet is balanced and the body free of yeast and toxicity. Hormone replacement therapy (HRT) is often recommended as standard procedure, despite the fact that it has potentially serious side effects, including increased risk of breast cancer.

Natural remedies include vitamins E and B complex, magnesium, evening primrose oil, ginseng, licorice, dong quai, black cohosh, damiana, and vitamin C. An extract of the wild Mexican yam called dioscorea is also proving helpful to many.

### Hyperactivity – see ADD                    DIM, YIR

### Hypertension – see Heart Disease      GN, AIR, TMR

### Impotence                                         YIR, TMR

Impotence, the inability for a male to maintain an erection, may be psychological or physical in nature. Check for poor circulation. Medications, alcohol, cigarettes, junk food, heavy metal deposits, and animal fats may contribute to this problem. Eat bee pollen, pumpkin seeds, royal jelly, vitamin E and zinc.

### Incontinence – see Bladder Infection and Kidney Stones                                            YIR, AIR

### Infection                                           AIR, YIR

Except for infections from cuts and wounds, infections indicate an inability of the immune system to render full protection. Infection has the potential for and often precedes numerous health problems from colds to gangrene to pneumonia.

Allergies and yeast overgrowth can overload the body's resources and set up a situation where infection can easily begin. Proper diet with fresh and whole foods rich in antioxidents are very important for protection, whereas caffeine, processed foods, and a toxic body give infection an advantage.

Very important for resisting and overcoming infection are vitamins A, C and B complex, zinc, selenium, and magnesium. Alfalfa, aloe vera, echinacea, garlic, ginger, golden seal, kelp, and uva ursi are helpful herbs.

### Infertility                                        YIR, TEI, DIM

The inability to conceive is becoming an increasingly

common problem. Poor diet, environmental toxicity, and yeast infection are all proving to contribute. We have seen many recover who have addressed these areas. Avoiding caffeine, smoking, alcohol, processed foods and eating fresh wholesome foods are very important.

Putting both man and woman on high dosages of the following supplements has "produced" at least one hundred babies born to otherwise infertile couples. Vitamin A 40,000 IU, calcium 1200 mg. with magnesium 600 mg., vitamin E 600 IU, selenium 300 mcg., zinc 40 mg., folic acid 800 mcg., and multiple minerals. It may take four or more months, but a friend of ours who is a nutrition counselor has over ninety baby pictures to prove that it works!

### Irritable Bowel Syndrome – see Crohn's Disease and Diverticulitis                                DIM, AIR

### Insomnia                                DIM, AIR, YIR, TMR

The inability to fall asleep or to stay sleeping on occasions is not abnormal, but if it becomes chronic such as in insomnia it may contribute to inefficiency in the body and even health breakdown. Check the category possibilities as well as find ways to alleviate stress. The amount of sleep required varies greatly with seasons and age and from person to person.

Reduce intake of chocolate, caffeine, salt, and smoked products. Helpful nutrients include minerals, B Complex, l-tryptophan and melatonin, also the herbs chamomile and valerian. Insomnia may also improve dramatically with regular exercise.

### Kidney Stones                                DIM

While some people tend to form kidney stones more readily, I believe they are greatly related to diet. High animal protein, caffeine, and chocolate increase stone-forming tendencies. The key supplement is magnesium. Also vitamin C (it does not cause kidney stones), B complex and vitamin A.

An old home remedy for helping to pass painful stones during an attack is to drink beer. It enlarges the urethra and allows stones to pass.

### Laryngitis AIR, YIR

This inflammation of the larynx, the upper voice box, often begins with a tickling sensation at the back of the throat. Soon after, there may be a hoarseness of the voice followed by a loss of voice. Sometimes the condition is not particularly painful so the person tries harder to use the voice which simply aggravates the situation. Letting the voice rest is important for faster healing.

The problem usually results from a yeast or bacterial infection for which antibiotics are not helpful. It may also be brought on by excessive use of the voice, especially while under stress, by allergies, or inhaling irritating substances.

Consuming fresh fruits, vegetables, and unsweetened juices, as well as avoiding sugar, caffeine, dairy products, smoking and alcohol speed recovery. Vitamin C 500 mg each hour, vitamin A 30,000 IU per day, garlic, zinc lozenges, chamomile and echinacea are natural therapies. Gargling with tea made from licorice root may also be helpful.

### Leg Cramps DIM, YIR

These involuntary contractions or spasms of a leg or foot muscle occur most commonly at night when legs are cool or have poor circulation. It is often referred to as a "Charley horse." If it occurs in the day time or while walking, it is more apt to be serious. The most probable causes are poor mineral balance, especially a shortage of calcium, magnesium and potassium.

Poor circulation is also a contributing factor which may be helped by vitamins E, A, D, B6 and B complex. A diet rich in dark green leafy vegetables and alfalfa are helpful. In addition to the above, vitamin E may be helpful for restless leg syndrome as it improves blood circulation.

## Lupus

*Description:* Lupus is a chronic inflammatory autoimmune disease. This means that the body is in effect attacking itself. About 80 percent of those affected are women. There are two types of lupus: systemic lupus erythematosus (SLE) which affects the joints and organs of the body, and discoid lupus erythematosus (DLE) which is a less serious skin disease. Both types may come on gradually or very suddenly and may flare up or go into remission.

DLE which affects the skin begins with a rash that forms over the nose and cheeks and neck. It tends to leave facial scars and discoloration. This is why it has been named lupus after the Latin word for wolf. The sun often causes the rash to flare up.

SLE patients complain of pain in joints. The kidneys may also be affected.

*Background considerations:* The cause of lupus is unclear but may be due to a virus that causes the immune system to attack the body's own tissue and organs. Various factors may cause a person to be more susceptible to SLE. Among these are stress, viral infections, immunizations, root-canal work, and silver mercury dental fillings. Certain drugs such as procaineamie, hydralazine, anti-convulsants, penicillin, sulfa drugs and birth control pills may also be predisposing factors.

*Possible disease category:* AIR, YIR

*Home/folk remedies:* Eat sardines or salmon three times per week.

*Natural therapies:* Check for food allergies. Concentrate on building up and normalizing the immune system; consider a detoxification program.

*Diet:* Avoid salt, pork, beef and high fat dairy products. Eat whole foods, fresh vegetables, fish, and fish oils as in sardines and essential fatty acids as in flax seed oil, sunflower or safflower oils. Avoid alfalfa sprouts.

*Nutrients:* Fresh carrot and celery juice; vitamins E, C, A, B complex, B12, B6, pantothenic acid, selenium; evening primrose oil, flax seed oil, OPC; also digestive enzymes, especially hydrochloric acid.

*Herbs:* Aloe vera, comfrey, yarrow, licorice, echinacea, golden seal.

*Other:* Dr. Jonathan Wright believes that 100 percent of SLE patients have food allergies. For optimal recovery, these must be determined and addressed.

### Lyme Disease                                                    AIR

This disease is transmitted by a tiny tick which is carried by the whitetail deer. It may also be transmitted by white-footed field mice, jackrabbits, and carried into homes by pets. The bites are at first hardly noticeable but later appear as a rash. It can develop into flu like symptoms, headache, stiff neck and backache, even nausea and vomiting. Enlarged spleen, irregular heart rhythm, arthritis and brain damage can occur.

Since it is difficult to detect, if there is any possibility of its occurrence, tests should be taken. Resistance and recovery require a strong and active immune system. All efforts should be taken to strengthen the immune system, among them, excellent diet, garlic, green drinks, vitamin C 6,000 mg, vitamin A, E, zinc, minerals, echinacea, golden seal, and acidophilus.

### Macular Degeneration – Eye Problems                     YIR

Macular degeneration and other age related vision problems seem to be an almost inevitable problem of aging. Vision can however, be considerably preserved by proper diet and certain herbs. Caffeine has a negative effect on vision, as do chemicals in processed foods.

Vitamins A and D are especially important for night blindness; vitamins C and E help to minimize vision problems. Carrot juice is excellent as are herbs such as eyebright and golden seal. One doctor reports that the vision of 50 percent of his cataract patients was restored by proper nutrition.

## Migraines – see Headache          DIM, TEI, YIR

## Mononucleosis – see Chronic Fatigue Syndrome
AIR, YIR

## Morning Sickness          DIM, YIR, TMR

The nausea, upset stomach, and sick feeling which many women experience during the early stages of pregnancy is caused by a rapid change in hormones. The feeling may be aggravated by odors from cooking or from poorly ventilated rooms.

Be sure there is an adequate supply of nutrients, especially minerals, and B vitamins. Sometimes lemonade is helpful; in other cases, ginger or additional protein may bring relief. Morning sickness does not indicate any problem with the developing fetus and usually disappears after the first several months of pregnancy. See Chapter 15.

## Motion Sickness          DIM

Those suffering from motion sickness experience symptoms such as headache, nausea, upset stomach, and sometimes vomiting. It relates to motion and may be experienced when traveling in a car, train, boat or plane. It seems to be the result of the brain receiving conflicting messages from the inner ear's balancing mechanism and the eyes.

Get as much fresh air as possible, take ginger tablets before traveling as well as B complex and magnesium. These may also be helpful when motion sickness is beginning. Magnets on wrist bands seem to give relief to cruise ship passengers. Straps hung from car bumpers to release static electricity have not been proven, but many insist that they limit motion sickness. If it works, why knock it just because we can't understand it. Besides, we used it when our children were little and they all survived!

## Multiple Sclerosis – MS

Multiple sclerosis is a chronic degenerative disease that causes the deterioration of the protective coating of the nerve cells (myelin sheath) in the brain and spinal chord. It varies in severity and may disappear for periods of time and return intermittently.

Symptoms vary from person to person, and may range from fatigue, visual problems, and numbness to speech disturbances, dizziness, bowel and bladder problems, lack of physical coordination and loss of balance.

*Background considerations:* Correcting nutrient deficiencies, and dealing with food allergies have been found to slow down or even eliminate the symptoms of multiple sclerosis.

*Possible disease category:* YIR, AIR  May be diet related.

*Home/folk remedies:* Vegetarian whole food diet.

*Natural therapies:* A strong active immune system is most crucial.

*Diet:* Fresh fruits, vegetables, nuts and grains. Definitely avoid all dairy products, caffeine, fats, processed foods, and alcohol.

*Nutrients:* High in all vitamins and minerals; also lecithin, evening primrose oil, CoQ10, and green drinks.

*Herbs:* Echinacea

*Other:* Check for possible sensitivity to mercury from fillings. Body detoxification may be helpful. For a nutrition program which has proven successful see *Healthy Steps*, Chapter 7.

### Muscle Cramps - see Leg Cramps                    DIM, YIR

### Nail Problems                                      DIM, TMR

The fingernails are protectors of the nerve rich finger tips. To some therapists they are windows to the health of the body. Common problems are often due to nutrient deficiencies. Opaque white bands on brittle nails may indicate a protein deficiency. This along with vitamin A and calcium deficiency results in slow growth.

White spots may indicate a shortage of zinc and vitamin B6. Thick nails may indicate circulation problems. Try spirulina for a good source of protein. The herb, horsetail is rich in silicon and is very helpful for nails and skin.

### Nausea – see suggestions for Morning Sickness and
### Motion Sickness                      DIM, YIR, AIR

### Nose Bleeds                                    TMR, YIR

Nose bleeds usually occur from a scratch, severe blowing of the nose, or a blow to the nose. It may also be instigated by blood thinning medications.

If nose bleeds occur frequently or are difficult to stop, increase vitamin K intake for better clotting. Vitamin K is found in kale, kelp, alfalfa, and in all leafy green vegetables. After a nose bleed apply vitamin E oil or aloe vera gel in nostril. Increased vitamin C intake is also helpful.

### Obesity – see Chapter 6 on Weight Control
### DIM, TMR, TEI

### Osteoporosis                                DIM, TMR

Osteoporosis is the gradual loss of bone mass resulting in increased fractures, loss of height, pain in the hips and back and curvature of the spine. The major cause is a lack of calcium. This may be due to a dietary deficiency or a poor capacity to absorb calcium. Other contributing factors may be a lack of exercise, lactose intolerance, copper deficiency and reduced estrogen in menopausal women.

It has been shown that the standard diet of processed foods, sugar, carbonated drinks, caffeine, high protein, and salt consumption is a major reason for the high rate of osteoporosis. Excess protein prevents calcium from being absorbed by the kidneys. Some health researchers believe that the number one cause of osteoporosis is the consumption of animal products. ( See page 108.)

A fresh whole foods diet, high in calcium, magnesium, phosphorus, vitamin C, and vitamin D is excellent for prevention and treatment of this problem. Good natural sources of calcium are kelp, kale, nuts, seed, oats, seaweed, tofu, broccoli, and wheat germ.

### Parasites                                    TMR, YIR

Parasites are numerous organisms that feed and live off the human body. Some such as lice, ticks and fleas live outside the body, whereas many more, from long tapeworms to microscopic protozoa, make their home in the body. They probably affect three out of five people and play a significant role in frustrating the health and sapping the vitality of their hapless hosts. They can so overtax the immunes system that it has little reserve for the normal challenges necessary to maintain body protection.

It is becoming increasingly evident that parasites lie at, or should we say "work" at the base of much disease and health breakdown. Many long standing health problems have quickly subsided when parasites were dealt with. An adequate body detoxification must also address the problem of parasites. (See Chapter 12 for more on detoxification.)

For prevention of parasites, it is important that hands be washed frequently, all raw foods be washed in salt water and cooked foods be cooked thoroughly. Deworm pets regularly, don't let them lick your face, and don't walk barefoot where they walk.

Herbs, such as black walnut leaves and hulls, raw pumpkin seeds, cloves, and grapefruit seed extract are natural treatments for parasites.

### Parkinson's Disease

*Description:* Also called shaking palsy, Parkinson's disease is a degenerative disease affecting the nervous system. Symptoms include, slowness of movement, muscular rigidity, involuntary tremors, excessive salivation, impaired speech, and staring facial expressions. A unique characteristic is a pill-rolling movement of the thumb and fingers. Mental activity is not impaired.

*Background considerations:* Symptoms seem to relate to an imbalance of two chemicals in the brain, dopamine and acetylcholine. These substances control muscle function by transferring messages between nerve cells.

Some therapist believe that dealing with resentment and unresolved anger, or the need to control others may help some people deal with the symptoms of Parkinson's.

There is no known cure for this disease. L-dopa, or levodopa is a drug often used but not without significant side effects, and should not be taken with vitamin B6. Vitamin B6 alone may be just as effective. Natural therapies can greatly slow down the progression of this disease.

*Possible disease category:* AIR, YIR Check for and deal with allergies, yeast and toxicity.

*Home/folk remedies:* Fasting with raw juices.

*Natural therapies*

*Diet:* Eat fresh fruits and vegetables and avoid processed foods, dairy, meat, and alcohol.

*Nutrients:* Calcium, magnesium, vitamin C, B complex, B6.

*Herbs:* Garlic, passion flower.

*Other:* Hydrogen peroxide therapy may be of some benefit.

### Periodontal Disease                    DIM, YIR

Also referred to as gingivitis in its early stages, this is an inflammations of the tissue that surrounds and supports the teeth. In the advanced state, pyorrhea, the gum is deteriorating and the teeth may break loose. Symptoms are red inflamed gum tissue that bleeds easily, usually without pain.

This disease is the result of poor oral hygiene, poor nutrition, sugar, smoking, drugs, and excessive alcohol.

Fresh and whole foods, proper brushing and flossing, multiple vitamin mineral supplements, CoQ10, and apple cider vinegar are healthy natural treatments.

### Premenstrual Syndrome – PMS             TMR, YIR

A hormone related disorder that affects menstruating women one to two weeks before the menstrual cycle begins. Symptoms may include mood swings from depression to fits of anger, cramps, headache, breast swelling, and insomnia.

PMS may be related to candidiasis, food allergies, thyroid imbalance and poor nutrition. When these areas are addressed, the problem may improve dramatically. The herbs, dong quai, blessed thistle, raspberry leaves, evening primrose oil, and squaw vine are also good for PMS.

### Postpartum Depression                                    YIR, AIR

After pregnancy, the woman's body undergoes considerable hormonal and other changes. Also, during pregnancy her body gave generously to the developing infant, and often short-changed itself. This along with the added stress and responsibility can become a near overload leaving the new mother depleted, exhausted and sometimes depressed.

Replenishing the mineral supply is important, as is B complex. Following the suggestions similar to those for chronic fatigue syndrome may help to prevent or greatly reduce the stress of this critical time of life.

### Prostate Problems

Common to at least one third of all men over fifty, enlargement of the prostate is known as prostatitis or benign hypertrophy of the prostate. The prostrate a small donut shaped organ of the male reproductive system surrounds the urinary outlet and restricts the flow of urine. Symptoms are reduced flow of urine, frequent urination and difficulty in starting and stopping urination.

*Background considerations:* While prostatitis is common and usually benign, one should be aware that prostate cancer is very common. Any unusual change, swelling, pain or blood in the urine should be immediately and carefully checked.

*Possible disease category:* AIR, YIR While there is no definite known cause for prostate problems, yeast and allergies may be contributing factors. Coffee, colas and processed meats may contribute to the problem.

*Home/folk remedies:* Raw pumpkin seeds. Regular exercise.

*Natural therapies:* Drink lots of fresh clean water.

*Diet:* Eat fresh fruits and vegetables, nuts and raw seeds. Avoid animal products, especially fats.

*Nutrients:* Zinc, 60 mg daily, vitamin E, bee pollen.

*Herbs:* Saw palmetto, marshmallow, juniper berry, golden seal and uva ursi.

*Other:* Walking is a helpful excellent exercise. Hydrotherapy may be helpful.

### Psoriasis                                                    YIR, AIR

Psoriasis shows up on the scalp, wrists, elbows and ankles, as a reddened rash covered with overlapping silvery scales. It results from a pile up of skin cells that have replicated too quickly. It can be activated by stress, surgery, illness, sunburns, or infections. Although there is no known cure, nutrient supplements, controlling yeast and dietary adjustments may be helpful. Only the body can cure itself.

Vitamins A, C, E, B complex, folic acid, pantothenic acid, evening primrose oil, and zinc are helpful. Herbs such as dandelion, goldenseal, and sarsaparilla are also useful. A low fat, high fiber diet with lots of fresh vegetables and fruits is also helpful for recovery.

### Restless Leg Syndrome – see Leg Cramps     TMR, AIR

### Rheumatism – see Fibromyalgia          AIR, YIR, DIM

### Shingles                                                   YIR, TEI

These painful blisters are a kind of left over adult form of chicken pox, which may have been dormant for many years. Low immunity, stress, yeast overgrowth, or poor diet may give this latent virus the opportunity to resurface.

Nutrients may help. Begin with B complex to encourage proper nerve function. Add vitamins C, A and E, as well as a good multivitamin mineral formula. Protein, especially vegetable protein is useful; I suggest spirulina, brown rice, grains and fruits. In addition, the herbs licorice, peppers, and parsley should prove helpful.

### Sinus Infection/ Sinusitis – see Infection      AIR, YIR

### Sore Throat          AIR, YIR

The mucous membranes at the back of the mouth and throat are very sensitive and subject to irritation and infection. Bacterial infections, allergic reactions, and extremely hot or cold drinks are just a few of the onslaughts the throat is subject to. A sore throat is often an extension to the common cold. If the immune function is strong, a sore throat may last a few days otherwise it could last a week or more.

Deal with a possible yeast problem, take vitamin C, 500 mg per hour, garlic, acidophilus, green drinks, and zinc lozenges. Sore throat is one of the very rare ailments I have experienced personally. My remedy, bathe the throat with garlic oil from capsules, or eat a fresh garlic sandwich at bedtime. I also take vitamin C every hour, at times using the tablets as lozenges. I have never had to miss a speaking engagement due to a sore throat.

### Sudden Infant Death Syndrome (SIDS)      DIM

The sudden death of an apparently healthy infant that cannot be specifically linked to a particular cause. It is the primary cause of the death of children, about 7,000 per year in the U.S., between ages 1 week and 1 year.

Medical experts have put forward some possible contributing factors. Among these are, a possible magnesium deficiency, and/or a vitamin C deficiency. These can be alleviated by being breast-fed by a mother who uses supplements, or giving the child supplements directly.

There are also those who believe that there is a correlation between SIDS and infant vaccinations. This is vigorously denied by medical authorities, but it merits serious consideration. See Chapter 15 and the bibliography for more information.

### Tonsillitis

Tonsillitis, occurring mostly in young children is an

inflammation of the glands of lymph tissue located on either side of the entrance to the throat. The tonsils which are intended to trap and fight infections become over whelmed when virus and bacteria take advantage when the body's resistance is low. With each reoccurrence, scar tissue remains and a cure becomes more difficult, so, it is important to begin a natural therapy as soon as symptoms appear.

*Background considerations:* A possible reason for this infection may be a diet too high in carbohydrates (sweets), and low in protein and other essential nutrients, especially vitamin C. Symptoms include, sore throat, white coating, painful swallowing, headache, earache, bad breath, fever and chills. In past years, surgical removal of tonsils was considered standard procedure. It's the only hospital experience I ever had or hope to have! By now we realize that tonsils do play a defensive role in the body and surgical removal is recommended only if absolutely necessary.

*Possible disease category:* AIR, YIR Allergies, yeast and diet are usually factors

*Home/folk remedies:* Gargle with warm salt water. Tie a sock around your neck over night.

*Natural therapies*

*Diet:* Avoid all sweets, pastries, white flour and dairy products. Drink clean water, fruit and vegetable juices and eat steamed vegetables and broth.

*Nutrients:* Vitamins C and D, zinc, B complex, vitamin E and acidophilus.

*Herbs:* Chamomile, echinacea, garlic, goldenseal.

*Other:* Rest and drink plenty of fluids.

## Ulcers

The term ulcer usually refers to a damaged lining of the gastrointestinal tract. An ulcer of the stomach is called a peptic ulcer and in the lower stomach it is referred to as a duodenal ulcer. Mucus protects the walls of the stomach from its acid contents. Once the lining is damaged, healing may be slow and difficult.

*Background considerations:* High stress, especially during eating, constant use of aspirin and steroids or other medications as well as smoking may contribute to stomach ulcers.

*Possible disease category:* DIM, YIR, AIR

*Home/folk remedies:* Drink freshly made cabbage juice, one liter per day for ten days.

*Natural therapies*

*Diet:* Avoid, fried foods, dairy products, caffeine, animal fats and carbonated drinks.

*Nutrients:* Vitamin E, iron, B complex, vitamin K, zinc and acidophilus.

*Herbs:* Aloe vera juice, cayenne, licorice, chamomile, and slippery elm.

*Other:* Recent studies indicate that ulcers may be due to a bacteria called Helicobater pylori and if this bacteria is treated, ulcers will be permanently healed. You may wish to check this with your doctor.

### Urinary problems – see Bladder Infection and Kidney Stones                                                    YIR, AIR

### Vaginitis                                                                    YIR

A burning, itching inflammation of the vagina. It may be caused by bacterial or yeast infection, especially if antibiotics, a vitamin B deficiency, hormonal problems, excessive douching, or intestinal parasites are present.

Treat the yeast condition as indicated earlier, use garlic as a natural antibiotic, take vitamins A, B complex, D and E. Add apple cider vinegar to water for a sitz bath.

### Varicose Veins                                                            DIM, YIR

Abnormally large swollen veins appearing most often in the legs. The valves in the veins which hold the blood between heart beats break down and the blood "pools" and swells the vein. Long-term sitting or standing without moving may contribute to this condition. If this is part of your job, take a few moments to stand and walk at least each hour. Vitamin E and vitamin C are most important for healing. See also information on hemorrhoids.

### Vitiligo                                      TMR, DIM

When the skin can no longer produce melanin, a skin pigment, white patches with dark boarders appear. This ailment called vitiligo may indicate a thyroid problem. It sometimes can be alleviated by good nutrition and supplemental PABA 300 mg, B complex and pantothenic acid 500 mg. Essential fatty acids are also helpful.

### Warts                                          YIR, AIR

Let's give the toads a break, they do not cause warts! Warts are the result of a virus and range in size from a pin head to a pea. They seem to prefer fingers and hands but will settle for anywhere. The virus is very contagious and spreads by touch; it enters scratches or scrapes. Sometimes warts go away on their own. If they are surgically removed, the virus may remain and cause new warts to grow.

Be sure yeast is under control and the immune system is strong. Vitamins C, A, B and E, and zinc are most important. Home remedies abound. Crushed garlic cloves, rubbing a raw potato or applying castor oil all lay claim to fame. Here's one more: In the morning apply a paste of vitamin A; in the afternoon add a drop of castor oil; in the evening apply a drop of lemon juice, and good-bye warts!

Have a healthy, happy wart-free day, eh!!!

# BIBLIOGRAPHY

Atkins, Robert C. *Dr. Atkins' Nutrition Breakthrough*. New York: Bantam Books, 1981

Balch, James F., M.D. and Phyllis A. Balch. *Prescriptiom of Nurtitional Healing*. Garden City Park, NY: Avery Publishing Group Inc. 1990

Berger, Stuart M., M.D. *What Your Doctor Didn't Learn in Medical School*. New York: William Morrow and Company, 1988

Bland, Jeffrey. *Nutraerobics*. San Francisco: Harper and Row, 1985

Bragg, Paul C. and Patricia Bragg. *Healthful Eating Without Confusion*. Santa Barbara, CA

Bragg, Paul C. and Patricia Bragg. *The Natural Way to Reduce*. Santa Barbara, CA 1992

Cheraskin, E., W. M. Ringsdorf, and J. W. Clark. *Diet and Disease*. Emmaus, PA.: Rodale Books, 1968

Clark, Linda. *Get Well Naturally*. New York: DevinAdair Co.,1965

Crayhon, Robert, M.S. *Robert Crayhon's Nutrition Made Simple*. New York: M.Evans and Company, Inc., 1994

Crook, William G. *The Yeast Connection*. New York: Random House, 1987

Diamond, Harvey and Marilyn. *Living Health*. New York: Warner Books, 1987

Erasumus, Udo. *Fats and Oils*.Vancouver, BC: Alive Books, 1986

Gottschall, Elaine. *Food and the Gut Reaction*. London, ON: Kirkton Press, 1987.

Hoffer, Abram, and Mortin Walker. *Nutrients to Age Without Senility*. New Canaan, Conn: Keats Publ., 1980

Jensen, Bernard, D.C. *Tissue Cleansing Through Bowel Management*. Escondido, CA: 1981

Kunin, Richard A. *Mega Nutrition*. New York: McGraw-Hill, 1980.

Kirschmann, Gayla J. *Nutrition Almanac Fourth Edition*. New York: McGraw-Hill, 1996.

Matsen, Jonn *Eating Alive*. North Vancouver, BC: Crompton Books, Ltd., 1987

Mendelson, Robert S. *How to Raise a Healthy Child in Spite of Your Doctor*. New York: Ballantine Books, 1984

Neustaedter, Randall. *The Immunization Decision*. Berkeley, California: North Atlantic Books, 1990.

Neustaedter, Randall. *The Vaccine Guide*. Berkley Ca.: North Atlantic Books, 1996

Pearson, Durk, and Sandy Shaw. *Life Extension -A Practical Scientific Approach*. New York: Warner Books, 1982

*Part Three* _____
*Health Problems and Natural Remedies*

Philpott, W.H. & Kalita, D. *Brain Allergies*. New Canaan, Conn.: Keats Publishing, 1980

Quillin, Patrick. Beating Cancer With Nutrition, Tulsa The Nutrition Times Press, 1994

Robbins, John *May All Be Fed – Diet for a New World.* New York: William Morrow & Co., 1992

Rona, Zolton P., M.D., *The Joy of Health*. Willowdale, ON: Hounslow Press, 1991

Royal, Penny C. *Herbally Yours*. Provo, Utah: Biworld Publishers, 1979.

Smith, Lendon. *Feed Your Kids Right*. McGraw Hill, NY. 1979

Thomas, John, *Young Again! How to Reverse the Aging Process.* Kelos, WA : Plexus Press, 1994

Virkler, Mark and Patti, *Eden's Health Plan – Go Natural!* Shippensburg, PA: Destiny Image Publishers, 1994

Walker, Norman W., D.Sc., *Colon Health: Key to Vibrant Health*. Prescott, AZ, 1979

Whitaker, Julian, MD. *Is Heart surgery Necessary?* Washington, D.C.: Regenery Publishing, 1995.

Wright, Jonathan B. *Dr. Wright's Book of Nutritional Therapy*. Emmaus, PA: Rodale Press, Rev. 1990

Yntema, Sharon. *Vegetarian Baby*. Ithaca, NY: McBooks Press, 1991

Zehr, Albert, *Healthy Steps to Maintain or Regain Natural Good Health*. Surrey, BC: Abundant Health Publishers, 1990

# Index

## A

A SED 90–92, 160, 209
Absorption 150
Acidophilus 56
Acne 214
Acquired Immune Dysfunction
 215
Activity Levels
 and food consumption 98
ADD 215
Adrenal Hormones 131
Age Spots 215
Aging 113, 129
AIDS 215
Air quality, Indoor 73
Air quality, Outdoor 72, 78
Alcohol 68, 120
Allergic Rhinitis 238
Allergies 120, 160, 204
 dairy 56, 98, 107
 testing for 109, 196
Alopecia 238
Aluminium 68, 69, 104
Aluminum 138
Alzheimer's 216
Amalgam Fillings 75
Amino Acids
 combining 111, 144
Angina 115, 120
Antacids 69
Antibiotics
 55, 56, 68, 181, 204
Antibiotics, Natural 204
Antibodies 50–51. See also
 Immune System
Antioxidants 159
 before conception 165
 to protect heart 129
Antiperspirants 68, 152

Arteries 106
Arthritis
 41, 72, 113, 115, 120, 151, 217
Aspartame 69, 205, 234
Assimilation 117, 150. See
 also Digestion
Asthma 120, 218
Athletes
 and protein 111
Attention Deficit Disorder 215
Autism 184, 218
Autoimmune Disease 160
Avocados 115

## B

Babies
 food for 177
 growth spurts 172
 importance of breast-feeding
 170
Baby Foods 177
Back Pain 219
Bacteria 158
Bacteria, Friendly 56
Bad Breath 219
Baldness 238
Barnes Test 206
Bathing 122
Bedsores 219
Beef 105
Bible 192
Bio-kinesiology 200
Bioflavanoids 134
Biotin 133
Birth Control 76
Birth Defects 132, 166
Black Currant Seed Oil 114
Bladder Infection 220
Blood Pressure 115
Blood Sugar 113, 142
Body
 as a whole unit 33–34, 49
 interfering with 54
 percentage water 119

 self-healing capacity 32, 90
 three phases of 117
Body Talk 58–59, 195. See
 also Pain: interpretation of
Boils 220
Borage Oil 114
Boron 138
Bowel 154. See also Colon
Bragg, Paul 109
Brain Development 115
Breakfast 117–118
Breast Infections 172
Breast Milk 115, 170
 supply of 172
Breast-feeding
 affect of caffeine 171
 and ear infections 232
 and medication 173
 and water intake 171
 difficulties with 171–172
 importance of relaxation 171
 let down 172
 nipple confusion 172
 nutrition for 171
 stopping 174–175, 176
Breathing, Deep 152
Butter 108

## C

Caffeine 70, 171
Calcium 134
 absorption of 113
 and protein 111
 from dairy 107–108
Cancer 221–222
 contributing factors
 68, 70, 113
 development of 160
 prevention of 55
Candida Albicans
 56, 165, 204, 222
 and infertility 165
Candidiasis 222
Candy 69. See also Sugar

Canker  223
Canola Oil  115
Carbohydrates  115–117
   digestion of  142
Carbohydrates, Complex
      143.  See also Complex
      Carbohydrates
Carbohydrates, Refined
      116, 143
Carbohydrates, Simple  143
Carpal Tunnel Syndrome  223
Cataracts  223
Celiac  208
Celiac Disease  223
Cell Division  160
Cell Phones  71
Cells, Mutant  160
Cellular Waste  150
Chemicals,
   in the workplace  69
   phyto-  See Phytochemicals
   testing of  62
   toxic  55
Chia Seeds  115
Chicken  105
Childbirth  168
Childhood Health
   root of problems  163
Children
   fussy eaters  180–181
   need for physical affection  169
   snacks for  178, 180
   vaccinations for  183
Chlorine  79
Cholesterol  109, 113, 224
   reduction of  115, 129, 142
Choline  133
Chromium  113, 136
Chronic Fatigue Syndrome
      78, 120, 225
Cigarettes  70, 166.  See also
      Smoking
Cirrhosis  226
Cleaning Products  70

Clothing.  See Fabric
Coenzymes  146
Coffee  120, 122
Cold Sores  223
Colds  226
Colic  182, 227
Colon  154
   constipation  71
   problems  108
Complex Carbohydrates  113
Computer Radiation  71
Conception  164, 165
Constipation  71, 227
Constitution, Physical  79
Contraceptives.  See Birth
      Control
Cooking Oils  104, 115
Cookware  69, 104
Copper  136
CoQ10  146
Corn  115
Crayhon, Robert  109
Crohn's Disease  227
Crystal Energy  140–141

D

Dairy  107–109, 182
   allergies  56, 98, 107, 109
   and calcium loss  111
   digestion of  56
Dandelion Root  147
Dandruff  228
Dehydration  120
Deodorants  69
Depression  228
Dermatitis  229
Detoxification  155
Detoxification,
   before conception  164
   need for  51, 80
Diabetes  69, 113, 229
Diaper Rash  230
Diarrhea  71, 231

Diet
   importance of  125
Dietary Principles  97–99
Diets  103
Digestion  56, 116, 150
   and sugars  113
   and water  123
Digestion Problems  106
Digestive Enzymes  145, 158
Diphtheria  183
Disability from birth  203
Disease Management  18–19
Diseases
   diet-related  40
   genetic  202
Diseases, "Incurable"  34
Distillation  121–122
Diuretics
   and pregnancy  167
Diverticulitis  231
Down's Syndrome  72
Dropsy  233
Drug Therapy
   dangers of  126
   dependency on  33, 47, 52
   development of  48
Dry Eyes  231

E

Ear Infection  232
Ear Piercing  139
Eating, Principles for Healthy
      97–99
Eczema  108, 115, 233
Edema  167, 233
EFAs.  See Essential Fatty Acids
Egg
   health of  164
Eggs  109–110
Electric Blankets  71
Electromagnetic Radiation
      71, 73, 165, 166
Elimination  117

Emphysema 233
Endometriosis 234
Energy
    from protein 110
Environmental Pollution 151
Enzymes 145–146
Epilepsy 234
Essential Fatty Acids
        106, 114–115, 129
Essiac 221
Estrogen 241
Evening Primrose Oil 114
Exercise 81
Exhaustion 111

F

Fabric, Synthetic versus Natural
        70
Fainting 235
Fast Food 72
Fatigue. See Chronic Fatigue
        Syndrome
Fatigue During Pregnancy 166
Fats 106, 114–115, 141
    unsaturated and saturated
        115
Fats, Hydrogenated 142
Fats, Monounsaturated 142
Fats, Polyunsaturated 141
Fertilization 164
Fertilizers 40
Fetal Growth 132, 166
Fever 182
Fiber 150, 154
Fibromyalgia 78, 235
Fish 105
Flanagan, Drs. Patrick and
        Gael Crystal 140
Flatulence 236
Flax Seed 114
Flax Seed Oil 104
Flour, Refined White 38, 69
Flu 237

Fluorescent Lights 72
Fluoride 139
    toxicity 72, 79
Folic Acid 132
Food
    combining 81, 98, 115–117
    for immune strength 161
    preparation 104–105
    principles for choosing 97–
        99, 208
    quantity and activity level 98
Food Allergies. See Allergies
Food Preparation 72, 76
Food Processing 38, 155
Free Radicals 115, 151, 160
Fruit 104, 116, 117
Fruit, Canned 104
Fungus. See Candida Albicans

G

Gallbladder Disorders 237
Gallstones 113
Garlic 204
Genesis 188
Genetic Disease. See Diseases:
        genetic
Germanium 139
Ginger
    and morning sickness 166
Gingivitis 251
Glucose 111
Glycogen 143
Goats Milk 174
God 188
Goldenseal 204
Gout 237
Grain 38
Grains 115
Grape Seed Oil 104

H

Hair Dyes 73
Hair Loss 238

Halitosis 219
Hamburger 106
Hay Fever 238
Headache 239
Headaches 108
Health Breakdown 201
Health Protection Act (Canada)
        34
Heart 129
Heart Burn 239
Heart Disease 29, 239
    contributing factors
        77, 108, 113
Heart Rhythm 123
Heel Spurs 241
Hemorrhaging
    during pregnancy 167
Hemorrhoids 241
Herbal Medicine. See Herbs
Herbs 49, 147
Hives 108
Holistic. See Body: as a whole
        unit
Honey 114, 174
Hot Flashes 241
Human Body. See Body
Hydrogenated Oils 115
Hyperactivity 69
Hypertension 120
Hyperthyroidism 205
Hypothyroidism 205

I

Ice Cream 74
Immune System 56, 203
    and water 123
    breakdown 75, 113
    operation of 50–51, 158
    response to cancer 160
    support of 50
    suppression of 50
Immunization. See Vaccina-
        tions

*Impotence  242*
*Incurable Diseases.  See
     Diseases, "Incurable"*
*Indigestion.  See Digestion
     Problems*
*Infant Formula  115*
*Infection  158, 242*
*Infertility  164–165, 242*
*Ingestion  117*
*Inherited Disease.  See Diseases:
     genetic*
*Inositol  133*
*Insomnia  243*
*Insulin  113*
*Interpretation of Pain.  See
     Pain: interpretation of*
*Interpretation of
     Symptoms.  See Symptoms:
     interpretation of*
*Intestinal Tract  56*
*Iodine  136*
*Iron  136*

*J*

*Jesus Christ  190*

*K*

*Kidney Stones  243*
*Kidneys  113, 153*

*L*

*Labor and Delivery.  See
     Childbirth*
*Lactobacillus Acidophilus and
     Bulgaricu  56*
*Lactose  56*
*Lactose Intolerance  107.  See
     also Dairy: allergies*
*Laetrile  132*
*Lappe, Frances Moore  111*
*Laryngitis  244*
*Leg Cramps  244*

*Legs
     restless  167*
*Lighting  72*
*Linoleic Acid  114, 115, 129*
*Linolenic Acid  114, 129*
*Liver  226*
*Love and Children  169*
*Lungs  152*
*Lupus  245*
*Lyme Disease  246*

*M*

*Macular Degeneration  246*
*Magnesium  134
     absorption of  113*
*Malnutrition  39*
*Man, the Three Parts of  186*
*Manganese  137*
*Maple Syrup  114*
*Margarine  74, 108, 115*
*Meat  74, 105–106
     and children  179
     preparation of  105*
*Meat, Processed  76*
*Medical System
     a monopoly  34, 57
     dependency on  28–29
     failure of self policing  31–32
     obsessed with symptoms  18*
*Medications  75*
*Medicine
     outcome based  24*
*Menopause  241*
*Mercury  75*
*Microclusters  140*
*Microwave Ovens  76, 105*
*Migraines  113*
*Milk.  See Dairy*
*Milk, Goats.  See Goats Milk*
*Minerals, Colloidal  140*
*Minerals, Trace  122*
*Miscarriage, Preventing  167*
*Molybdenum  139*

*Morning Sickness
     166, 167, 247*
*Motion Sickness  247*
*MS  108*
*Multiple Sclerosis  247.  See also
     MS*
*Muscle Cramps  167*
*Muscle Testing  200*

*N*

*Nail Problems  248*
*Nanocolloids  140*
*Nasal Congestion  108*
*Niacin  130*
*Nickel  139*
*Nose Bleeds  249*
*Nursing.  See Breast-feeding*
*Nutrient Depletion in Soil  40*
*Nuts  115*

*O*

*Obesity  83, 113*
*Oils, Cooking.  See Cooking
     Oils*
*Olive Oil  104*
*Omega-3  114*
*Omega-6  114*
*Organic versus Synthetic  57*
*Osteoporosis  108, 111, 249*
*Overweight  123.  See also
     Weight Control*
*Ozonation  121*

*P*

*PABA  132*
*Pain
     function of  46
     interpretation of  45.  See also
          Body Talk*
*Pain Relief  30*
*Pancreas  113*
*Pangamic Acid  132*

*Pantothenic Acid  131*
*Parasites  250*
*Parkinson's Disease  250*
*Periodontal Disease  251*
*Pharmaceutical Business*
  *profit motive  18,  29*
*Phosphorus  135*
*Phytochemicals  55*
*Phytonutrients  146*
*PMS  251*
*Polio  183*
*Pork  105*
*Postpartum Depression  252*
*Potassium  77,  135*
*Potatoes  116*
*Preconception  164–165*
*Pregnancy  165–166*
  *and cigarette smoke  166*
  *and EMR  166*
  *diet for  115,  166*
  *nutrients for  132,  167*
  *problems during  167*
*Premenstrual Syndrome  251*
*Prescription drugs*
  *danger of  126*
*Probiotics  56*
*Processed Food.  See Food*
  *Processing*
*Processed Meat.  See Meat,*
  *Processed*
*Profit Motive  18,  29*
*Prostate Problems  252*
*Protein  144*
  *alternative sources of  179*
  *and athletes  111*
  *and calcium loss  111*
  *complete  111*
  *excess  111*
  *for energy  110*
  *from vegetables  111*
  *needs  110–111*
  *with carbohydrates  115–117*
*Psoriasis  115,  253*
*Pumpkins  115*

*Pyridoxine  131*

*Q*

*Quacks, Medical  23,  26,  57*

*R*

*Raspberry Tea*
  *and childbirth  168*
*Relief of Pain.  See Symptomatic*
  *Relief*
*Respiratory Illness  108,  204*
*Reverse Osmosis  121*
*Riboflavin  130*
*Rice  116*
*Rice Syrup  114*
*Robbins, John  107,  108*
*Root Canals  77*
*Rubella  183*

*S*

*Safflower  115*
*Salad Dressings  104*
*Salt  69,  77*
*Science*
  *purpose of  23,  27*
*Selenium  41,  137*
*Senile Dementia  216*
*Sexual Promiscuity  77*
*Shingles  253*
*Shortening  115*
*Shute Brothers  24*
*SIDS  254.  See also Sudden*
  *Infant Death Syndrome*
*Silicon  140*
*Sinus Congestion.  See Nasal*
  *Congestion*
*Skin  152,  157,  204,  214*
  *itchy during pregnancy  167*
*SLE  245*
*Sleep  78,  198*
*Smoking  165.  See also*
  *Cigarettes*
*Snacks  180*

*Sodas.  See Soft Drinks*
*Sodium  135*
*Soft Drinks  69,  78,  120*
*Soil Nutrient Depletion  40*
*Sore Throat  254*
*Soul of Man  186*
*Soybean  115*
*Sperm*
  *health of  164*
*Spirit of God  190,  192*
*Spirit of Man  187*
*Spiritual Growth  192*
*Spirulina  111*
*Starches  116*
*Stomach.  See Digestion*
  *acidity  113*
*Stress*
  *and vitamin C  73*
  *damaging effects of  73*
*Stretch Marks  167*
*Sudden Infant Death Syndrome*
  *184,  254*
*Sugar*
  *negative effects of  113–114*
  *substitutes  114*
*Sulphur  137*
*Sunburn  132*
*Sunflower  115*
*Supplements  81,  125*
  *dangers of  126*
  *need for  126*
*Sweeteners  175.  See also Sugar*
*Symptomatic Relief  30,  47*
*Symptoms,*
  *interpretation of  47*
*Synthetic versus Organic  56*
*Systemic Lupus Erythematosus*
  *245*

*T*

*Taste  197*
*Tea  120*
*Teeth.  See Tooth*
  *Fillings;  Toothpaste*

*Teflon  104*
*Thankfulness  100*
*Thiamine  130*
*Thyroid  205*
*Tonsillitis  255*
*Tooth Fillings  75*
*Toothpaste  72*
*Toxemia  167*
*Toxins  123,  150,  206*
  *affect on nursing infants  171*
*Trace Minerals.  See Minerals,*
  *Trace*
*Tree of Life  188*
*Triglycerides  113*

*U*

*Ulcers  108,  255*
*Ultra Violet Light*
  *for water purification  121*
*Unsaturated Fatty Acids  129*
*Urination  123*

*V*

*Vaccinations  51,  159,  183–*
  *184*
*Vaginitis  256*
*Vanadium  140*
*Varicose Veins  113,  256*
*Vegetable Protein  111*
*Vegetables  104*
  *cooking of  104*
*Vegetarianism  106,  111,  131*

*Vitamin*
  *A  128*
  *B Complex  130*
    *depletion of  113*
  *B1  130*
  *B12  131*
  *B15  132*
  *B17  132*
  *B2  130*
  *B3  130*
  *B5  131*
  *B6  131*
    *and morning sickness  166*
  *C  80,  133–134*
    *and morning sickness  166*
    *and stress  74*
  *D  128*
  *defined  127*
  *E  129*
  *F  114,  129*
  *K  56,  129*
  *P  134*
*Vitiligo  257*

*W*

*Walnuts  115*
*Warts  257*
*Water  78*
  *and breastfeeding  171*
  *and kidney function  153*
  *function as a solvent  119*
  *ice  123*

  *in the body  119*
  *purification methods  121*
  *retention  123*
  *substitutes for  120*
  *when to drink  122*
*Weaning  174*
*Weight Control  83.  See also*
  *Overweight*
*Wheat, Processing of  38*
*White Flour.  See Flour, Refined*
  *White*
*Wholistic.  See Body: as a whole*
  *unit*

*X*

*X-rays  79*

*Y*

*Yeast  204.  See also Candida*
  *Albicans*
*yeast  68*
*Yogurt  174*

*Z*

*Zinc  138*

also from Dr. Albert Zehr

# *Healthy Steps*

## to maintain or regain natural good health

## Simple, understandable, practical, useful.

Albert Zehr, Ph.D. Nutrition, shares practical suggestions and specific natural programs that have helped thousands step out of ill health.

### HOW TO:

Take healthy steps out of · fatigue · indigestion · insomnia · forgetfulness · Candida Yeast Infection · obesity · heart disease · Epstein-Barr Virus/Chronic Fatigue Syndrome · and more.

After explaining the backward steps that brought us into health failure, Dr. Zehr shows us how to get into step with our body, so that any health conscious individual can help himself to take healthy steps towards natural good health.

Abundant Health Publishers
151-10090 152nd St., Ste. 531, Surrey, BC V3R 8X8

604-930-2326